FIRST TIME DENTIST

Your Detailed Roadmap to Buying the Practice of Your Dreams

First Edition

Adam Heim

Disclaimer

© Adam Heim 2016

This book is written for informational, educational, and entertainment purposes only as they relate to the business of dentistry, not the practice of dentistry. Neither Adam Heim nor ATH Capital LLC or its Members or affiliates are dentists, medical experts, or experts in any area of the field of healthcare. No part of this book shall be construed as advice on how to practice in the field of dentistry, other medicine, or the broader field of healthcare.

The viewpoints provided are opinion based on Adam Heim's own experience, experiences may vary. Always seek out legal or financial advice from a licensed professional before acting on any information.

While we try to keep the information up-to-date and correct, there are no representations or warranties, express or implied, about the completeness, accuracy, reliability, suitability or availability with respect to the information, products, services, or related graphics contained in this document for any purpose. Any use of this information is at your own risk.

No part of this work may be reproduced or transmitted in any form or by any means, electronic or mechanical, including photocopying, recording or by any information storage and retrieval system, without the expressed written permission from the author.

*"All of our dreams can come true,
If we have the courage to pursue them."*
-Walt Disney

TABLE OF CONTENTS

First Time Dentist 1
Table of Contents 4
Acknowledgements 7
Foreword 9
Introduction 11
    My Story: 12
    Some Inspiration 15
Chapter 1: Lifestyle Design 17
    Why? 19
    Developing Your Vision 20
    Bringing it All Together 23
    Financial Lifestyle 24
    Are you meant to be an owner? 26
    Recap 30
Chapter 2: Building Your Team 31
    Building Your Team 32
    Process of Selecting Advisors: 34
    Interviewing Lawyers 37
    Interviewing Accountants 38
    Surveying Lenders 40
    Interviewing Bankers 42
    Recap 42
Chapter 3: Getting Started 43

    Determining a Location 43
    Lease vs. Own... 46
    Commercial Real Estate 49
    How Much Will It Cost Me? 50
    Creating You Practice Profile 52
    Practice Search Tactics 53
    Recap... 56

Chapter 4: Preliminary Due Diligence 57
    Location Analysis.. 59
    Mystery Shopping... 63
    Non-Disclosure Agreement 70
    Preliminary Data Request 72
    Data Request Checklist: 73
    Practice Financials.. 75
    Recap... 85

Chapter 5: Due Diligence 86
    Financials and Valuation Overview... 87
    Practice Valuation... 89
    Real Estate 91
    Engaging Your Team 93
    Site Visit 96
    Evaluation of Facilities 99
    Chart Evaluation... 102
    Business Operations Evaluation 104
    Staff Evaluation and Salaries... 110
    Spouses & Family Members: 111
    Employee Manual: 112
    Bringing it All Together 113
    Recap.. 115

Chapter 6: Negotiations 116
    Making an Offer 118
    Letter of Intent... 126
    Finalizing the Agreements 130
    Next Steps 132
    Final Iterations 134
    Recap.. 135

Chapter 7: Closing... 136

Pre-Closing Checklist	137
Setting the Stage	145
Pay and Job Security	146
Benefits	147
Closing Day – What to Expect	148
Chapter 8: Post Closing	**149**
How to Survive Your First Week	154
Living Life and Improving Your Practice	155
Conclusion	156
Final Thoughts	**158**
About the Author	**161**
End Notes	**162**

ACKNOWLEDGEMENTS

My wife, Amy - Of course I must first thank my wife Amy, without whom this book would not have been possible. She has taken me on quite a few adventures following her many 'visions' in the past few years, and I look forward to the adventures for a long time to come. I am always thankful for her on-going support of my, sometimes outlandish ideas in the pursuit of success.

My Parents (Tom and Sandy) – I also can't publish a book without also thanking my parents, I learned many of my greatest qualities from each of you – discipline, an eye for detail, persistence and humility. I thank you for absolutely everything you have (and have not) given me in life.

My In-Laws (Gary and Vicki) – I hesitate even using the term 'in-laws' as it has such a negative connotation, much the opposite of what I feel for Gary and Vicki. I am certain that without your never-ending help we would not be where we are today. Whether it was home projects, last-minute dental hygiene substitution, inputting insurance forms, or fixing a broken dishwasher – you guys truly rock! I couldn't ask for better neighbors or a family to have joined.

My Wife's Mentor (Dr. Marvin Cohen) – While I did not have the day-to-day interactions with Dr. Cohen as my wife did during her residency program, I did hear second hand about the wonderful accomplishments, endless leadership qualities, and timeless wisdom. He helped us buy the dental practice with his 'pay it forward' attitude – always ensuring the next generation has more knowledge than the one prior. His determination to pursue a residency program, his keen understanding of business, and his love for teaching will have forever changed the course of our lives and will far outreach even his wildest dreams. I too hope to 'pay it forward' with this book. To quote Doctor Cohen's mantra: 'Fortune Favors the Bold'.

Sheri Kay ([SKY Dental Practice Coaching](#)**)** – I'm not sure where we would be without having met you. You have changed my / our perspectives on practice ownership, leadership, life, and even my diet! Thank you!

All the people I missed – we are far to blessed to have the time to list every wonderful person we have met along the way, but I am certain that those not mentioned know that I/we appreciate their support.

Adam Heim

FOREWORD

When I was in dental school, my primary focus was to pass my boards, not harm any of my patients, and graduate. Little did I know that the one-hour practice management class, that I slept through in the back of the room, would be information I would actually need in the future.

In my last year of "D" school I was more concerned with my patients showing up in the clinic so I could seat my last graduation requirement. As opposed to writing business plans or learning about practice transitions. That seemed so far off in the distance... until, it came, sooner than expected.

After dental school graduation, I began a one-year residency program, two hours away from my now husband, Adam. During this year I did some soul searching for what the next step of my career. While we were trying to figure out where we would move after we got married, an opportunity too good to pass up became available in my hometown.

Adam and I jumped head first into this acquisition with little assistance to guide the way. To say I am lucky to be married to my husband, Adam Heim, is a huge understatement. Throughout the entire transition to practice ownership, he was my steadfast anchor. Adam handled the lawyers, the brokers, the accountants, the insurance companies, the appraisers, the bankers, the mounds of paperwork, and the never-ending phone calls.

Outside of Adam, my residency director, Dr. Marvin Cohen, served as our only real mentor and trustworthy source of information. He gave up his Saturday mornings to review numbers and talk about buying/owning a practice.

The purchase deadline came and went and after the champagne glasses were empty... business ownership, and its frustrations, was all ours. The first year of practice ownership and of our marriage was a time of tension and stress.

Let's face it, I was just trying to prepare a crown correctly and do a quadrant of composite without someone looking over my shoulder. Now, I had a staff of seven grown women with more combined years of experience than I will have in my entire career. I never would have made that first year without the unwavering and undying support of Adam, my husband.

He may not be able to prepare a #30 chamfer margin, but he is more than confident and versed in practice transition. He was very disheartened throughout the purchase process when we were unable to find credible, trustworthy and unbiased information related to practice transactions. Thus, he has dedicated the next chapter of his life to helping dentists take action towards elevating their careers and becoming business owners.

They say without blood, sweat and tears, the end result is less than deserved. Believe me in saying that every ounce of our own blood, sweat, and tears has been invested in this practice. Adam would love to be able to save you the agony of walking alone in that experience. Dentistry is challenging enough, let alone trying to buy a practice alone.

Now, he continues to walk alongside me as I am into revamping my practice vision and thriving in practice ownership. He can hold his own in a conversation about comprehensive dentistry, bite splint fabrication, and lab communication on an implant case. He is a one of a kind man of integrity that when he puts his mind to something, a goal is achieved.

Because he is my husband, I can attribute his support to being married, but it extends much deeper than that. My husband is dedicated in offering the same support to you. Think of this book as having your own personal Adam to help walk alongside you in your journey. Reach out to him as he would be more than happy to help you along the way.

Remember - the goal is to thrive, not just survive. Welcome to the next chapter of your life... PRACTICE OWNERSHIP.

-- Amy L. Heim
Amy L. Heim DDS LLC
Portsmouth, Ohio

INTRODUCTION

"The point of maximum danger is the point of minimum fear"
- Will Smith

First and foremost, I would like to thank and congratulate you on buying this book. This small step will be, hopefully, the first of many subsequent actions which will one day be known as your 'career'. On the cover of this book, you will find my mission statement, which is to "Inspire practice ownership, through action."

Action is a key theme in this book and in many of the books I have read by entrepreneurs, leaders, or visionaries. Action is what differentiates entrepreneurs from 'wantrepreneurs'. Action can be big. Often you see the great visionaries of our generation idolized for their focus on disrupting the world.

However, actions that change the world, or your career path, do not have to be audacious tasks. Sometimes the simple things like picking up a certain book, calling a broker, making contact with a dental lender, etc. are the small actions which snowball into your eventual dream. I hope you find this book to be inspiring. Just remember, inspiration without action is just day-dreaming.

In the meantime, please do not ever hesitate to look me up on FirstTimeDentist.com should you have any thoughts, questions or comments. I intend for this site to be the 'go to' resource for anyone looking to buy a dental practice.

My Story:

I spent the better part of my life in Cleveland, Ohio pursuing a career in business. As with many things in life, you follow opportunities as they present themselves. So here I am writing a book about buying a dental practice? I can assure you, this was never part of my wildest dreams in college. However, I have found that some of our greatest accomplishments in life are born out of the culmination of your own life experiences crossed with your passions.

I graduated with a degree in Finance and Economics in 2008 from a small university in Cleveland. My task, leading up to graduation, was of course to find a place of employment. I entered the workforce, as many others did in 2008, facing the most dismal economy since the great depression.

Every day, it seemed, another financial institution was collapsing. Major employers were laying off people in droves, and I decided that this was the perfect time to get into banking. Needless to say, finding a job was quite difficult, let alone finding one in an industry (banking) which was actively imploding. Through persistence and determination, I finally landed that internship and it was one of the most exciting moments of my career.

After I spent the better part of a year at this internship, and had been turned down for one internal position, I decided to pursue opportunities at different banks. My formal career really started when I moved to Columbus, Ohio in 2010 to pursue the first full-time / permanent position that had been offered to me after graduating. My manager at the bank in Cleveland unexpectedly left and moved to Columbus, only to call me up and offer to bring me along for the ride (note that networking and connections are <u>crucial</u> in the business world).

I then spent the next decade working in various roles in the retail bank, everything from setting interest rates on multi-billion-dollar portfolios (talk about nerve-racking for a 23-year-old), to studying demographics for branch placement, and building financial models for Real Estate transactions, and working on several Mergers & Acquisitions. I had a great job with a great income doing interesting work. I had dreams of becoming a successful bank executive, continuing to move up the corporate ladder when my career trajectory changed, dramatically.

When I first met my wife, I was awestruck by her beautiful eyes and the fact that she almost tackled me when we first met (I went for a cordial hand-shake but she insisted on something reminiscent of a bear hug).

Beyond our natural connection and ease of conversation, I was also amazed at her overflowing positivity, ambitious dreams, and outgoing nature. She was still in dental school and already had here eye on a practice that may be coming up for sale in her hometown.

Time went on, we got engaged and then had to start thinking seriously of where we would live. I was from the Northeastern part of Ohio, four and a half hours away from her home time, yet we met in the middle of the state. At first, I had considered the thought of following her down to Southern Ohio, only to quickly dismiss it as unrealistic as it would take me too far away from my own aspirations.

I'm not sure if it was just the onset of time, which has a funny way of distorting your previous doctrines, or the allure of realizing a long-forgotten dream of mine (to live life in a smaller and/or rural town). Regardless, I eventually came around to the idea of moving away and helping to pursue her dream of being a business owner.

Next, we then began one of the most stressful periods of our lives up to that point. In addition to living at other ends of the state (she was pursuing a residency for a year) while we were planning our wedding, she was also simultaneously pursuing a prospective practice. By the time our wedding day came around, we had already negotiated the majority of the purchase and had a closing date set after our wedding.

We then moved out of our two apartments and into a third, took a honeymoon a few weeks later and bought the practice, all in less than <u>eight weeks</u> after getting married. Thankfully, I was able to keep my job working the majority of the week from home. This provided one of the only sources of stability and reliable income, while we were learning the ropes of her newfound career.

<u>One week</u> before she closed, she sat on the couch, looked over at me with a tired, almost sick look in her face and proceeded to describe to me how she had thought we had 'bitten off more than we could chew.' Here we were, about to make the largest investment of our lives and she *now* she is questioning everything we've done over the past year? The thousands of dollars we had already spent, the hours of traveling, working with lawyers, the endless calls with lenders, *now* after all that she's concerned whether we made the right move? To say that I was not flooded with emotions (fear, anger, sadness, compassion, concern, etc.) is an understatement. Quite honestly, I didn't know what to do, who to talk to or how the hell we were going to make it. Despite this, we marched onward into the great unknown.

The majority of the first year of her owning her practice (and our marriage) was basically a blur of uncertainty and weariness. The long days/nights, steep learning curve and lack of support created an undesirable and often challenging home life. I do chuckle a bit when I hear couples recall their romantic honeymoons followed by a first year of marriage bliss. I'm not laughing out of distain for them, but more from a place of envy as we spent our first 365 days in haze of complicated emotions. We spent the precious minutes leading up to our honeymoon negotiating contracts and reading dental magazines from the beach in Mexico. My tale does have a happy ending, in that, we managed to get our feet under us (a bit) and we've learned tons about running a business and marriage.

I wanted to share this story with you for two reasons – first, I wanted you to understand that I/we have been in your shoes and know the emotional challenges involved with buying a practice. Second, I wanted you to understand my motivation for putting together this book and my website. When I reflect on our experience now I often wonder – did it have to be that hard? The answer is 'no'. I hope to provide you with the right level of knowledge, preparation, and support so that you can navigate the process with confidence and conviction.

All of this, has led me to the creation of FirstTimeDentist.com. I will speak more to the benefits later, but I hope that I can provide you with the tools, resources, insights, services and support in pursuit of your dream practice.

I thank you deeply for your purchase of the book and look forward to your thoughts, feedback and success stories.

Some Inspiration

Before we get started in helping you find the practice of YOUR dreams, just a few words of (hopeful) wisdom...

I lead an inspired life. It is one of my greatest blessings, that I can become intrigued, passionate, and knowledgeable about a random topic all because of a well-worded speech, a well-positioned article, or a deep conversation.

Why do you care about my inspirations in life? I think this book will, if nothing else, demonstrate to you that anything is possible in life. I follow quite a few business leaders on social media and there seems to be a few common themes in running a successful business.

The first is that no one is going to hand it to you. It will require grit and hard-work that others are not willing to attempt. As Howard Farran states in his book Uncomplicate Business[i] –

> *"Work like no one else will for the first 10 years of your career, so that you can live like no one else does for the rest of your life".*

Second, no one ever succeeds by happenstance. Successful businesses set a goal, build a process/product, and develop a system and a strong level of discipline in pursuing this goal. If the goal is stale, they change it, if the process doesn't work, they fix it, and if they get distracted then they re-align themselves – it is a constant system of checks and balances. For more on this topic, read the Checklist Manifesto[ii] by Atul Gawande.

Lastly, successful businesses are built through authenticity and compassion. You must have both a mission for what you want to change in this world, and a certain level of compassion, whether that's for your patients, customers, employees, vendors, or the guy walking down the street. If you're mission is to get rich, you will eventually fail in the larger picture. Do not be successful in just your financials, work hard to ensure that all aspects of your life are enriched through this process – faith, family, experiences, creativity, passions, and profession.

The remainder of this book is going to focus very intently on the exact steps you need to take and questions you need to ask, to ensure you are buying the right practice for you. This process is, at times, far from inspirational. As you go through this process you will have ups and downs, times where you say 'I can't wait to be an owner' and times where you say 'I can't wait for this to be over'.

When this happens, just keep revisiting whatever inspires you. There has to be something deep down that inspires you to purchase a dental practice, otherwise you wouldn't be reading this book! Keep that close, protect it, and use it when you hit your bottom, because you will, everyone will hit a bottom at this process at some point or another. Do not let fear of failure stop you from succeeding, fear is a mindset one that is malleable and controllable.

Will Smith[iii] describes, in an online motivational video, his experience in sky-diving. He talks about the amount of fear he had the night before, on the ride to the launch site, on the plane ride up, etc. He builds the anticipation, fear and apprehension up – right until that moment that he jumps out of the plane and let's go of the fear and is overwhelmed with a feeling of bliss. He says two profound things about his change in mindset on his emotions involved in this experience:

"You realize that at the point of maximum danger is minimum fear"
...and "God placed the best things in life on the other side of terror"

CHAPTER 1: LIFESTYLE DESIGN

"If you have built castles in the air, your work need not be lost; that is where they should be. Now put the foundations under them."
- Henry David Thoreau

Hello and welcome to the first chapter on your journey to purchasing a dental practice!

The purpose of this chapter is to mentally prepare you for the tasks that lie ahead. Purchasing a practice will be a stressful endeavor, full of unexpected outcomes and challenges that you will likely never face again in your life (this is probably a good thing!). Regardless, before you continue, we need to ensure that you have properly explored your own passions, desires, and goals – in order to set you up for success (and sanity), post-closing.

The biggest mistake that I personally believe a new dentist can make when purchasing a practice has really nothing to even do with the practice. Sure, there are obvious pitfalls of buying a practice (always have an accountant and lawyer helping you, fact-check and do not assume, etc.). What most of these checks-and-balances are attempting to avoid, however, are consequences which are more short-term in nature. My concern is that you, the dentist, need only be happy and satisfied with your practice purchase for years to come. Long-term wealth, health, and enjoyment will never follow, if you are unsatisfied with 'Why' you bought your practice.

In the coming pages, I will teach you the ins-and-outs of how to think about long-term planning. While I'm sure you're anxious to jump into the nitty gritty of the practice purchase process, I want you to take a step back first and work on the 'soft stuff'. Take the time to truly contemplate the following pages. Do so in a quiet room when you have time to think, without distractions. An understanding of yourself will become one of your biggest assets as you begin to live out your dream.

Why?

If you haven't already heard of Simon Sinek, you'll want to check out his TED talk Start with Why [iv]. In it, Simon discusses a core concept that most businesses fail to grasp – 'Why'. If you're answer to the question of "Why do you want to be a practice owner?" is that you want to 'make lots of money' or 'work only four days a week', or 'be your own boss' – note that you have been warned!

Making money and looking forward to a 3-day weekend is not going to comfort you when you're firing your first employee, when you're working nights or weekends to improve your practice, or when you lay up in bed at night worrying about how in the hell you're going to complete some procedure or task tomorrow.

Your 'Why' needs to be something more grandiose, driven by more than just dollars-and-cents. Money is an outcome, so is happiness, success, etc. Developing your 'Why' (Vision Statement is part of the next section) will serve as an inspiration piece for your employees, your patients, and in the hard times – even you.

Starter Thoughts / Exercises:

1. Ask yourself, not the topical self, but your core, your soul – Why do I want to buy a practice? What about it excites you? What about it scares you? What will your friends and family say?
2. Consider the type of environment you will breed (employees and patients) if you pursue this venture only for money.
3. Watch the Simon Sinek Ted Talk Start with Why.
4. Name a few companies who do have their 'Why' and others that do not.
5. List your 'Why' in a simple statement, it could be something like:

To serve my community; To build lasting relationships, to change people's lives – one smile at a time.

Developing Your Vision

The 'Why' is a simple test of your motivations. Next, we need to get more specific into What you want out of life. To do so, we need to develop a long-term Vision for both personal and professional lives.

Do not be modest, this is the time to take charge of your life and your future. I recommend taking an attitude which focuses on conquering your fears and approaching every challenge as an opportunity. One of my favorite quotes for this was taken from the book Who Moved My Cheese[v], by Spencer Johnson -

"What would you do if you weren't afraid?"

While child-like at times, it is an interesting read for the intellectually curious, as it focuses on human behavior and how, even in the simplest of ways, our attitude can shape the outcome of our lives.

Exercise 1: Personal Vision

---

1. Imagine you can live anywhere in the world you want – where would it be?
2. What would you do in this place, what would your hobbies, social life, or other interests consist of?
3. What are the core values that will drive the decisions?
4. Are you currently living a life that would fit these desires? If not, then why – what is holding you back?
5. Now, I want you to take all your answers and synthesize them into a single statement, here is an example of my Personal Vision:

I want to spend my life residing in the country, living a simple life. I want to cherish my close relationships, all the while enjoying the outdoors. I want to start/own several successful businesses over my career and help provide jobs to my community.

Exercise 2: Professional Vision

1. Would you be happier working alone or a group setting?
2. Would you like to mentor or work with an associate someday?
3. Are you interested in being a better business owner or clinician?
4. How would you envision your practice looking? Modern? Themed? Classic? Simple?
5. What types of dental organizations would you like to belong to? Everyone you come across? Local? None?
6. Do you have an office manager?
7. Who do your patients look like? Old? Young? Underserved? Affluent?
8. What do your employees look like? Do they run the practice making you the cruise director? Or are you a micro-manager, ensuring every detail is perfect?
9. Do you want to open/own multiple practices?
10. Do you want to run a high volume, low margin or a high margin low volume practice? Or somewhere in between?
11. How often do you take continuing education vs. travel vs. volunteer vs. relax?

Again, I want you to synthesize all your answers into a single statement, also taking into account your personal vision as well. An example of a statement may look like this (First Time Dentist's Vision Statement):

> "To CHANGE the way the dental industry buys and sells practices."

Remember, there are not many times in life where you can ask for anything and everything you want – but this is that time – take advantage of it! Be creative, witty, and inspired. For now, this will be your own personal treasure, but it could be something worth hanging on the wall at your future practice to serve as a reminder of where you are driving your life.

Now that you know the 'Why' (mission) and the 'What' (vision), you need to form the 'How' (your values). Values are the rules of the game, they keep you in-line when you begin to stray. Without values, you will do anything to achieve you mission, even if it means compromising your reputation, authenticity, morals, etc.

Again, please write these down along with your vision and why (see next section 'Bringing it All Together' for a template).

Exercise 3: Values

1. Think about the best and worst recent customer experiences you had. What was the defining factor in each? Communication? Respect for time? Feeling important?
2. Think about all the things in dentistry that you have heard, about that were ethically debatable, what feeling is elicited when you hear/see these stories? How would you have acted differently?
3. What piece of you/your reputation would you never give up for any amount of money?
4. As Warren Buffet[vi] once told his employees (I'm paraphrasing) – 'before you do anything of consequence, consider how this action would be viewed by your friends, family and neighbors; if it were plastered on the front page of the Sunday newspaper.' What actions or circumstances do you never want to end up on the front page?

Now let's build some guard rails around these feelings and how you will operate your business. I would choose 3-5 core values that you want to define both your business and you. Here is a short-list of values to consider, but by no means is this list all-inclusive:

Figure 1.1

Honesty	Pride	Humility
Integrity	Diversity	Discipline
Creativity	Innovation	Accountability
Relationships	Communication	Expertise
Personable	Philanthropy	Collaboration
Curiosity	Leadership	Community
Spirituality	Balance	Environment

Bringing it All Together

Now, bring all these aspects together into a one-page document. Lay it out however you want – it could be a beautiful document or a simple outline. Point is you want this document to be your foundation for how you approach business, life and al the challenges that are associated with each. You want this document to be your 'Opus', with content you can be proud of and happy to display and print. Maybe even include some inspirational quotes.

Putting this on a single page represents your commitment to everything written on it. You will be able to use this document as a guide post throughout the practice transition process, as well as your career. Do not skimp on thought here, this is you on a page – make it authentic.

Financial Lifestyle

Now that you know 'where' you want to go and 'why' you are embarking on this trip. Let's start to think about 'how' you are going to get there, financially. I would recommend creating a quick budget for your household. It doesn't have to be perfect or fancy by any means. If barroom napkins won't suffice and you insist on a spreadsheet - visit FirstTimeDentist.com to fill out a quick budgeting worksheet.

The output of any budget is really just an estimate as to how much cash you will have left over at the end of each month. Maybe consider doing a best case / worst case scenario to help you put some guardrails on the exercise. The key here is to be honest with yourself. If you want to spend money like it is going out of style, that is certainly your prerogative. While I have my own views of spending habits, that is a topic for another book I will someday write. For now, I just want to make sure that whatever you need out of a practice, financially, will be in the realm of possibilities.

Further, this exercise will come in handy when we get farther down the road on purchasing a practice. At some point, you will need to generate a financial Pro-Forma (projection) of what your practice will produce. If your number is significantly higher than what your potential practice is making in a given year, you either need to grow the practice, shrink your expenses, or search for a different practice which aligns closer to your financial needs.

Consider some of the following questions:

---

1. What type of car do I want to drive? Fancy sportscars, a mini-van, something in-between? How much would you spend?
2. Where do you want to live? Build a new home, buy a small home, fixer-upper, rent a home, rent an apartment?
3. How expensive is the city you want to live in?
4. Are you married/plan on getting married in the next 2-3 years?
5. Do you have or plan on having children in the next 2-3 years?
6. Do you like planning larger/exotic vacations?
7. How much do you regularly spend on the must haves (food, water, shelter) vs. the nice-to-haves (shopping and entertainment) vs. the REALLY nice to haves (European vacation, growing your craft beer or wine collection)?
8. What types of lifestyles do your closest friends and family live? Do you want more / need less?

You may also consider reading Tim Ferris's' book "The 4 -Hour Work Week" [vii]. In it, Tim describes how he has reinvented his life into a transient world traveler who manages multiple online businesses through the use of extreme automation. I will warn you – if you take what he says too literally, you will be disappointed in the book (as you can't automate or outsource root canals, no matter how hard you try).

The book does still serve as a great resource and inspiration for any budding business owner as he strives for efficiency in everything he does. Additionally, he talks at length about finding out how much you need to live and enjoy life. Once you hit that point, you should (according to Tim) minimize every second you spend on working. His point is that we should be trying to maximize how much we make per hour worked (by lessening the denominator), not how much we make in a year.

To do so, however, Tim describes needing to find your own monthly break-even point using his template. This is the point at which every dollar you make above/beyond is extra (and you're sacrificing your life to achieve).

Are you meant to be an owner?

Now that your personal and professional visions are complete, you need to ask yourself a serious question – are you meant to be an owner? The mentality of owning a practice is something that is not inherent in everyone. However, having the discipline to manage, intuition to lead, and determination to grind out the hard times – are the aspects of ownership which can be learned.

The challenge that many people face is described thoroughly in one of my favorite books E-Myth Revisited.[viii] In it, Michael Gerber discusses how most small business owners are actually technicians suffering from an entrepreneurial seizure. His point is that most business owners are really good at WHAT they are doing (i.e. – dentistry) but not at managing a people of technicians (i.e. – assistants, hygienists, front desk).

The book is an excellent read and will help you understand the importance of being honest with yourself about whether you are truly a business owner or a technician who is having a moment of entrepreurial desires. Remember, these moments fade and then you find yourself at the office until 10pm on a Tuesday night, doing some menial task. You need these entrepreneurial desires to extend beyond moments – you need them to come the deepest parts of your soul.

Below is a list of questions that you should consider before taking a leap into practice ownership. For each question, I've also included a few reasons why the question is important. Consider each carefully as you explore each of these concepts. Additionally, he discusses the importance of having 'systems' (i.e. – checklists and operating procedures, not IT systems) in place in a business.

Question 1: Are you easily discouraged when things do not go as planned?

While this will happen clinically, wherever you go, you will be surprised as to just how many things go wrong on a daily basis. In the first two years of my wife owning her practice, they lost power, water (twice), a patient had a heart-attack in the parking lot, and a car slid out of control and almost took out the corner of the building (also the room which my wife, an assistant, and a patient were working in at the same time). Let alone the multitude of small errors that occur every day. Every day will present its share of challenges and opportunities – you need the demeanor to be able to shake these events off and 'keep on trucking'.

Question 2: Are you willing to be accountable, for everything that occurs inside your practice?

One thing that I always remind my wife is that nearly 100% of the issues, communication challenges, and upsets that occur in her practice, is her fault. It is her fault because every time something bad happens – you, as the owner, need to be thinking of a way of stopping that issue from ever happening again in the future. You may even find yourself taking the blame for incidents in which your staff failed to perform correctly. You need to ensure that your pride will not be a barrier to accepting and correcting issues.

Question 3: Do you have a desire to learn more about business, financials, management?

Improving yourself clinically is certainly important, however unless you manage and grow your business – you will find yourself constantly trying to 'catch-up'. What gets measured is what gets improved. I recommend looking at financial statements on a monthly basis, completing an annual budget, and requesting that each of your employees enter in data into some type of tracking tool. This will give them ownership and reinforce to them that you are watching each of their individual performance levels.

Question 4: Create a list of all the types of self-doubt, insecurities, or situations that make you uncomfortable. How many of these do you think you can conquer? How many will (very likely) show up in your practice ownership tenure?

I want you to list out every one of your weaknesses here – do not take any shortcuts. Everyone has weaknesses about self-image, clinical abilities, ability to communicate with patients, ability to manage others, discomfort discussing money, fear of isolation (quite common in solo practices). By writing it out, you're acknowledging your vulnerability which, with continued exposure and effort, will desensitize your mind to the discomfort of each item on the list.

It is also very important that you try to relate each of these to items to a scenario that you will likely face once in practice. If being yelled at by a patient makes you uncomfortable, then play this scenario out in your head, over and over again. How would you react? What would you say? By doing this, you're mentally preparing yourself for the day in which this scenario is presented.

In his book The Power of Habit[ix] Charles Duhigg describes a similar approach taken by Gold Medal Olympian Michael Phelps. Of particular interest, is the story of how he would mentally (and physically) prepare for events by swimming in the dark. The reason was that if there were ever to be a goggle malfunction, then he would be completely prepared. You guessed it, it did actually happen to Michael during an Olympic race. His goggles filled with water and knew exactly how many strokes he had left and was able to not only win the race but also set a world record. All because he was mentally prepared for a very unique situation.

Now, if you truly do not have any weaknesses (you can't think of one!?) then I want you to stop reading this book and first go read the book Ego is the Enemy[x] by Ryan Holiday. You should also follow it up with the TED talk by Brene Brown called The Power of Vulnerability[xi]. And even if you do decide to keep reading, these two links (the latter being a free YouTube video).

Take this portion seriously and do not kid yourself. If you truly hate detailing with employees, accountants and lawyers – do not torture yourself with practice ownership. Some people are meant to be owners and some are not. Just like some people are meant to be Teachers and not Dentists. There is nothing misaligned with wanting to pursue a career in dentistry and take on none of the management responsibilities. Owning is a business is a lifestyle and we need to make sure it matches you and your visions.

Question 5: What will you enjoy most about being an owner?

Do you want to inspire patients to change their habits? Project leadership qualities onto your employees? Help your employees achieve financial goals? Or do you like the ability to constantly challenge your performance whether clinically or financially? On a day-to-day basis, what is going to make you smile and think 'yes, I made the right decision'?

FIRST TIME DENTIST

Recap

I hope this chapter helps spur some thoughts and deepen your understanding of yourself, your dreams, and your future.

Buying a practice can be one of the greatest and most challenging aspects of your adult life. So, I strive to make certain that you are fully prepared for the commitment you are about to pursue. Do not doubt your ability to do this, because that's why I designed this course. I will help you through every step of the process from looking, to buying, negotiating, and closing.

That said, if you've completed this chapter and you're worried that you're 'Why' may not be aligned with ownership, or that you lack the fortitude to just 'make it happen' – I would seriously caution you on pursuing a practice at this time. Keep in mind – this is a journey of a lifetime, no one says you have to start this journey now. If you prefer to take on less responsibility, maybe an associateship, clinic, or working for a larger chain of practices is a more desirable at this time – you can always revisit the idea later!

CHAPTER 2: BUILDING YOUR TEAM

"None of us is as smart as all of us" – Ken Blanchard

The next step in the process is to begin surrounding yourself with professional advisors to help you navigate the technicalities of purchasing a practice. Not only will these individuals help you to close on a practice, but they will likely be part of helping you run your business for years to come.

In this chapter, I stress the importance of a systematic approach to locating, interviewing, and decisioning each of your advisors for several reasons. I have provided a survey form (FirstTimeDentist.com) as well as a specific list of questions to ask each of these individuals. The bottom-line is that we want to ensure you select a group of advisors who are ready and able to help you. I want to help you avoid some of the mistakes I made in this process like not asking enough (or the right) questions.

Choosing your team should be one of the first things that you do prior to actually searching for a practice. Having the team already in place will allow you to avoid the unnecessary stress of trying to find an advisor at the last minute, or even worse, selecting the wrong advisor simply to get the deal inked.

I would like to reiterate this point, pursuing a practice without a lawyer and an accountant (at a minimum) is not only foolish, it is reckless. It will behoove you to start working with them early. There is a concept that my wife and I discuss often called CODB – 'Cost of Doing Business', and unfortunately you have to spend money to make money.

Building Your Team

I believe strongly that in order to execute anything in life, you need a game-plan. Thus, I have created a list and standardized approach for choosing the advisors you will need to carry you through the process of purchasing a practice.

First, however, I wanted to give a list of the primary and secondary advisors and a brief description of what they will do for you in this process...

Primary Advisors:

Lawyer – assist with Letter of Intent (LOI), advice on laws pertaining to opening/running a dental practice in your state, review and give legal guidance on all contracts, assist in negotiations, and business insights.

Accountant – should provide insight into how the business is currently operating (financially), how it will operate when you take over, as well as reviewing your personal situation to assist the lawyer in the formation of the best legal entity. Taxes should be an afterthought!

Lenders – I found it helpful to make connections with several lenders prior to the purchase – they were a wealth of information and very willing to meet and provide any help they could (yes, because they want to sell you a loan). While it may benefit you to working with the same bank that you're borrowing from, it is not a requirement.

Bankers – small business bankers can also be a great addition to your team. Not only can they double as your lender (depending on the lending practices at their institution) but they literally spend their days working with solely small business owners – giving them a deep understanding as to how businesses succeed (or fail).

Secondary Team Members:

These are advisors which should definitely be included on your team, however finding them is not as urgent as finding the primary team members.

Financial Advisor – can help you manage your finances (and protect yourself financially) in both your personal and professional life. You may wait until post close to find this individual, if you're not already working with someone.

Insurance Agent – will assist you in finding commercial lines of insurance for malpractice, property and casualty, but can also provide disability and life insurance.

Brokers – a broker can assist you in finding a practice (if you are struggling) and also representing you as a buyer. That said, I think there are some conflicting opinions on the value that brokers bring as they are typically focused on the sell-side. It may still be worth your time to do some research of your own and discover whether one can help you or not.

Payroll – at some point you will want to look for a payroll company. Some accountants also do payroll through their practices, but outside of that you have plenty of options. You can use Paychex or ADP (two of the largest companies) or you can always do an online search and find a few more local/regional companies.

Mentors – I strongly suggest contacting any friend, colleague, professor, attending doctor, or other individual whom has owned a practice in the past. My wife was very close with the director of her residency program and to this day I'm thankful for the advice he gave us as we wandered through this process in the dark.

Process of Selecting Advisors:

---

1. Using internet searches for your prospective state/area, attempt to locate 2-3 advisors in each category for the primary team members.

You may want to do the standard Facebook, Yelp, and website search for reviews or other insight you can gain about each person and their approach to their respective professions. Look for individuals who have the same style, approach, and feel to their practice, as you hope to have in yours.

---

2. Make initial contact with 2-3 advisors in each category.

I recommend starting with a simple e-mail to each advisor. The e-mail doesn't need to be fancy, simply stating that you're a dentist and you're looking to purchase a practice in the next XX months and are in need of some help. I would ask them if there was a time in the next week that they could have an introductory call / consultation. While this might seem passive aggressive approach (sending an e-mail) – I use it as a test. If someone doesn't e-mail me back within a few days...queue the buzzer! You will be transmitting quite a bit through e-mail (documents, financials, data, forms, etc.) so why do you want someone who doesn't answer you electronically?

---

3. Have a phone call (or in-person) conversation with each advisor.

I would give the advisor a time on X date in which they are to call you. This is, again, a test - did they end up calling on time (or close to)? I can't tell you how many sales calls I've had where the people have called be 15, 20, even 30 minutes late (or they are waiting for you to call them). I've ended up firing or ending our business dealings with every one of these people - if you can't be punctual for a new client, are you going to be punctual for an existing one?

4. Take studious notes during the call (specific questions to come in following sections).

Using the Advisor Survey Form to help you remember the conversation you had with each advisor as well as assist you in making your final selection. Take note of not only the specific content you discuss, but their demeanor as well – did the speak clearly and confidently? Were they distracted? Did you feel annoyed? Is this someone that you would share a beer with on a Friday after work?

The point is that this advisor you hire will be a part of your life in some way shape or form. While it is not a marriage, it should be someone that you at least respect and trust from the get-go. It doesn't have to be 'love-at-first sight', but it should be close.

5). You may way to end the call by asking whether they have any referrals for other advisors in the area.

It doesn't hurt to have advisors who already have a working relationship - IF (stressing the 'if') you end up liking those individuals as well. Do know that if the advisors are too wedded to each other and you end up needing to fire one, you may have some friction with the remaining individual.

6. After you have completed your interviews, take some time to review all the information you collected and make your decisions.

I would recommend sending an e-mail to each of the advisors you select, stating that you would like to hire them.

It might not be a bad idea to include the list of advisors you plan on hiring (along with contact information). This can be helpful in case one of them needed to reach out to another for a question (always great when you can get 'your people' talking amongst themselves and then coming to you with the results).

I would <u>not</u> recommend reaching out to those you do not want to pursue and letting them know. This will only cause additional probing as to why you went with one versus the other (if they are worth anything) – not worth your time, you followed your gut – now move on!

The scary thing is that of the ones you do not hire, I can almost bet that very few (if any) will ever reach out to you and ask for a status update – remember that point when you start practicing for yourself (...lost opportunity!). If they do call you back to check-in, respectfully let them know that you have chosen someone else and you will let them know if anything changes.

Again, please check out FirstTimeDentist.com for an Advisor Survey Form I created for you to help document, and then later, compare the candidates.

Interviewing Lawyers

Like it or not, your lawyer is your biggest asset in purchasing a practice, period. You will spend more time, money and effort with them than any other advisor through this process. Thus, ensuring you ask the right questions and can find a lawyer whom you trust and have a mutual level of respect is crucial. Lawyers can be intimidating to talk to but remember – they serve you. You are the client and they are they to make your dreams, whatever they may be, come true with little/no legal risks in the process.

Here is a specific list of questions I would ask when chatting with your prospective lawyers:

1. How long have they been practicing?
2. What are their practice specialties or areas of focus?
3. Have they ever helped a client in the practice transition process in the past? If not, have they helped clients buy other businesses (i.e. – not dental)? How many?
4. What is their advice for getting the most out of the due diligence process (process by which your completing formal research on a practice including financials, site visits, chart review, etc.)?
5. What is the range of cost they think they will need to charge in order to assist you in the practice purchase?
6. How much do they charge per hour?
7. Do they have a paralegal? How much are they per hour?
8. Do they require an up-front deposit?

My lawyer asked for a $5,000 deposit after I let him know I wanted to hire him – make sure you have full clarity of their expectations early on!

9. What is their typical turn-around time on document reviews/drafts?
10. 10 What do they see as the biggest risk in buying a dental practice?

Interviewing Accountants

I have spent many years trying to find a 'good' accountant. I have fired my share of them as many simply do not live up to the standards they set for themselves. While no set of questions or answers can give you a definitively foreshadow your experience, asking some very specific questions may help enrich your expectations.

You need to ask accountants lots of questions around process, deliverables and their approach to managing your financial risks.

Here are some questions I would pose to your accountants:
1. How many dental/medical clients do they have?
2. How much do you expect the accounting fees to be in a practice purchase? How much do they charge per hour?
3. Can you provide me with a detailed approach to how you would recommend we conduct due diligence?
   a. What specifically can I expect out of you during the due diligence process?
   b. Financial Statement Analysis?
   c. Income Tax Analysis?
   d. Written Write-Ups?
   e. Financial Projections?
   f. Practice Valuations?
   g. Other services?
4. Do they provide bookkeeping services? If so, how much do those usually cost?
5. Do they offer payroll solutions? Do they offer discounts if you did payroll through them?
6. Who exactly would you be working with on a day-to-day basis? Can you speak with them individually (if not the person on the phone)?
7. Sometimes you will be courted by the owner/higher-up accountants, but then work with the younger or more inexperienced accountants day-to-day, we just want to ensure that you trust both the company and your point of contact.
8. What types of actions can I take to avoid overpaying in taxes at the end of the year?
9. What is your approach to year-end tax planning? When do you usually start?

You want to take a mid-year view on taxes, do not work with an accountant who wants to wait until November/December – it makes it difficult to make changes at that point. Failing to plan for taxes (in a 'good' year) could cost you an (unexpected) lump sum in the thousands (or tens-of-thousands). Make sure your accountant is aligned with your annual progress (ideally include your financial advisor as well).

10. What do they see as the biggest risk in buying a dental practice?
11. How much working capital is needed (in terms of months' worth of expenses)?
12. Any other financial advice they can offer for managing your practice?

Surveying Lenders

As I mentioned, Lenders can be a wealth of information simply for the fact that they (like bankers) spend their days looking at financial statements and talking with business owners.

I actually started our practice purchase journey with a lender who was more than willing to send me a detailed e-mail and have a phone conversation. The key is, unlike your other advisors who will have a longer-term view – lenders are working off the here and now – they want to make the commission on selling you a loan in the next 3-6 months and are more energic about fulfilling your immediate needs.

Unlike your other advisors where you're trying to narrow down to only one individual/company, for Lenders, I recommend that you work 'in parallel' with multiple lenders (2-3). This does two things for you – first, it allows you to garner some competition for your business (hopefully giving you better deal terms). Secondly, it allows you the ability to have an instant back-up plan, should you get fairly deep into the deal, and one lender back-out unexpectedly (unlikely, but always possible).

Here is a list of questions I would consider asking a lender:
1. Does the financial institution specialize in medical or dental lending?
2. Would the lender require you to use SBA to get a loan?

SBA stands for 'Small Business Administration[xii]' loans. A quick summary is that these loans are backed by the federal government, allowing banks to take risks that might not have taken otherwise. This is a great thing for small business owners who want to open/expand their business, but do not have access to capital.

The downside of these loans is that they do carry some upfront fees which can be impactful, they take more time to process (since the government is involved) and they can carry a higher interest rate than other loans.

3. What are the typical deal terms for a dental loan?
    a. Term (in years)?
    b. Interest rate?
    c. Down payments? (shouldn't be any/much)
    d. Pre-payment/pay-off penalties?
    e. Interest only periods available?
    f. Are there any loan processing fees?
4. How much working capital would they recommend (compare to accountant's response)? Should this be a term loan or line-of-credit?

Think about working capital as your checkbook. It is money you have in the bank to pay your loans, utilities, employees, etc. If you buy a practice for $500k but only take a loan for

$500k – how will you pay you employees in 2 weeks? Capital / liquidity (having funds available) is the lifeblood of a business – without it, you're sunk.

5. Do they offer commercial real estate loans (where applicable)? If so, what are the terms of those (similar to question #3 above)?
6. Do they offer any discounts or benefits by bringing your operating account (i.e. – checking account) to their institution? What if you do your merchant processing through them (credit card processing)?
7. What type of paperwork will you be expected to fill-out?
8. What type of information will they require from you/selling doctor?
9. What is the process in which they follow to acquire a loan? How long does it usually take?
10. Do they offer pre-approvals? Is there a chance that the institution could back-out prior to closing (if pre-approved)?

I've heard some horror stories about dentists thinking they were 'pre-approved' for a loan, only to find that they were denied in the end and they had no backup plan. Beware of these gimmicks (with reputable names) and ask them point blank about their lending process.

11. What is their success rate that they see on dental practices that are purchased?
12. What is the biggest risk they see in buying a dental practice?
13. Do they require you to submit any on-going tracking post-close?

We had to participate in an 18-month reporting program which required inputting some 'key metrics to allow them to keep an eye on our progress. Honestly, it felt like more of a 'check-the-box' exercise than anything that provided real value – we never heard from the lender once, even though I later found mistakes in my own work...good intentions, just a bit clunky of process.

Interviewing Bankers

I decided to show two distinct sets of questions for Lenders vs. Bankers, as you may very well end up with an operating account (i.e. – checking) at one bank and a loan from another. For instance, we took out our practice loan with Bank of America: Practice Solutions[xiii], however they do not have a single brick-and-mortar location in the state of Ohio – thus we had to look elsewhere to do our day-to-day banking.

I do believe it is a good step, however to survey a few banks. While I would recommend a less intensive approach (likely do not need to complete full interviews like the other advisors) I would still recommend doing some research and reaching out to one or two intuitions. Again, you'll be amazed at who does not call you back.

Here are some questions to answer about a bank and their product sets:
1. Does the institution have a dental / medical-specific product set? If so, how do they differ from other Small Business Products?
2. Do they have bankers who work with medical businesses only?
3. What type of operating account is recommended?
4. Does the account have monthly fees?
5. Does the account have minimum balances?
6. Does the account offer an interest rate? If not, what products do?
7. What minimums or activity are required for those accounts?
8. Does the institution offer merchant services (credit card processing), payroll services, or lending services?
9. If you bring more/all of your business to the institution, do they provide you with any incentives?
10. How much working capital would they recommend to run your business?
11. What is the biggest risk they see in purchasing a dental practice?

Recap

Ok, I know you're just itching to get this process going and start doing some more fun stuff, like actually looking for a practice. Now that the ground-work is laid, we can begin to dive into the meat of the practice purchase process.

In Chapter 3 we're going to talk about the "Starting Your Search". We will provide you with lists of brokers to call, demographic resources, and a process on how to start collecting information about each practice you want to consider.

CHAPTER 3: GETTING STARTED

"Two roads diverged in a wood, and I – I took the one less travelled by and that has made all the difference" – Robert Frost

At this point, you've already done some soul-searching, designed your lifestyle, and begun to assemble your team. Now, this process is going to get fun...

Starting a practice search is no different than starting a search for a new home. You might have an idea of what you want, but you haven't sat down with your real estate agent yet and formally documented these wants. In this chapter, I want to help you create a specific set of criteria which you can use as an educated way of starting a conversation with a practice broker. Doing so will keep you honest (with yourself) about what you do and do not want out of a practice.

Additionally, I hope that by the end of this chapter, you're able to identify 2-3 locations on which to begin performing Due Diligence (formal process of investigating a practice).

Determining a Location

Determining where you want to practice can be one of the biggest challenges in this process. Let's be honest – this is a HUGE decision! A quick search online yields an interesting sample of statistics – the average American moves 8-12 times in their life (depending on your data source). So how are you ever going to be able to predict the general area where you want to spend the rest of your life (and be happy living there)?

Bottom-line is, you aren't...there is no way of truly understanding where you should live for the rest of your life. Or where your current (or future) spouse will want to live, where you will want your kids to go to school, etc. Or when you will suddenly decide that you should have bought a practice on the beach instead of the desert.

However, I hope that you can use the outcomes of the Lifestyle Design chapter to help you choose an area where you will at least be happy for the next 10 or so years. After that, you'll (hopefully) have your practice loan paid off and have the freedom to either continue practicing in this same area or sell the practice and go wherever life takes you.

Key Questions to Ask Yourself:
1. Do I want to live close to where I grew up?
2. Do I want to live close to where my family or friends live?
3. Do I have any proximity restrictions (non-compete) from a prior work arrangement (associateship or otherwise)?
4. Where does my spouse want to live?
5. What type of area do I want to live in? Urban, Suburban, Rural?

Demographically, you should also understand the area in which you plan on practicing. If you're planning on practicing in the area you grew-up in, or have lived in for an extended time, the demographics are probably less of a priority. However, if you are only generally familiar with the area you want to practice, or it is complete new, you must understand the demographic in this area.

While there are certainly 'better' areas to practice than others, the crucial outcome here is that you understand if your practice profile fits the area. If you are looking at buying a high-end aesthetic practice in a low-income area – you may be misaligned. Similarly, on the purchase of a bread-and-butter low cost/low expense practice that is located in a super-high-income area, may be misaligned as well.

Below are a few metrics I would recommend reviewing for your search area(s). I would recommend comparing three geographies, for example you could pull data for where you live now, where you grew up, and where you want to practice. This should give you a few comparison points to understand the different socio-economic profiles of each area.

Key Demographic Variables:

1. **Total Households** – you want to understand the number of households that live within a reasonable drive-time (this can differ by area, ask yourself 'how far/long would I drive to visit a dentist?'). This is, essentially, your 'market' that you will be trying to capture.

2. **Household Growth** – while quite a few areas in the Midwest (where I reside) have become accustomed to stagnating or slightly declining population, your big concern here is whether there has been a noticeable decline in recent years or is projected for the near future.

3. **Family Size / Number of People per Household** – depending on your target market (young singles vs. families) you will want to understand this metric to ensure your target area/practice is correctly positioned.

4. **Median Household Income** – knowing your patient profile is important (as mentioned above) – compare the Median Household Income to that of your state.

5. **Unemployment Rate** – as unemployment increases, the likelihood that monies will be spent for dental work is likely to tail-off, you want to be in an area that has reasonable unemployment rates vs. your state. Also, good to note, who are the major employers in the area, have new companies come to town? Are existing companies at risk for leaving?

6. **Number of Dentists per Capita (person)** – I would visit the ADA's site and look for competitors within a reasonable distance to get an idea of the number of competitors. Usually 2,000 is quoted as being the 'line in the sand' whereby more than 2,000 people / dentist suggests a better competitive dynamic for you.

There are a multitude of sources that will provide you insights on demographics. Below are a few that you can consider, some free and some range from cheap to expensive. As always – you do get what you pay for with demographics. Do make sure you weigh the need vs. the cost – if you grew up in your target area and have lived there for 30 years, you are likely to have a deep level of understanding of the demographics.

Free:
1. ESRI Business Analyst Online[xiv]– ESRI is the world's leading provider of mapping software and demographic data. They offer a 21-day free trial of their Online demographic data (relatively straight forward to use). I would start with this tool to get all your free information. Also, this tool could be something to invest in, longer term, when considering your marketing strategy.

2. City-Data[xv] – one of the easiest and simplest sources for demographic data on the internet (that I have found thus far), that said – they do not have a complete list of the variables shown above.
3. U.S. Census Bureau[xvi] – the underlying source of most demographic data in the country, however combing through their data can be a bit more time intensive.

Not Free:
1. ESRI 'Canned' Report[xvii] – ESRI is the industry leader in GIS software (mapping) and has a very reasonable product for around $50, if you are just looking for the bare minimum. It won't solve all the world's problems, but the data will give you a brief overview, in a clean format, at a fair price.
2. Dentagraphics[xviii] – of course, if you do not want to do the leg-work to look-up and understand the demographic information presented, you can utilize the Dentagraphics tool for a fee ($300-$500 depending on the report type). As usual, you get what you pay for – Dentagraphics offers a superior product compared to the rest of the options. I would recommend using their services if you are extremely unfamiliar with the area(s) you are considering. Additionally, they offer some added value in the form of social media research (who is using social media / digital advertising and to what extent).
4. Doctor Demographics – while I preferred the sample reports from Dentagraphics over Doctor Demographics, I wanted to provide you with the resource anyway, in case you find more value in their output. They likely offer more data in their reports, however Dentagraphics has much better visuals and an online tool which can be manipulated by the user.

Lease vs. Own

Another major consideration is whether you would prefer to own or lease your building. Note, that I said 'prefer', since this process is one giant negotiation, you never know where you may end. Regardless, here are some things to consider and ask yourself in either scenario.

Leasing Considerations:
1. Provides flexibility, in case you want to relocate your office someday in the future.
2. Does not tie-up capital in the building, may allow you to have a higher level of cash-flow.
3. Rent is considered a business expense (which reduces taxable income) whereas with a mortgage payment only the interest is considered a business expenses (therefore you're technically getting taxed on your principal payment, even though that cash is not available to you.
4. Shifts much of the maintenance responsibility to the Landlord.
5. Likely an easier path to closing financing with a bank.
6. Requires that you typically give-up significant control over building signage, alterations, improvements, needed maintenance, etc.
7. Term/optionality risks do exist – your landlord can (at some point) kick-you out, leaving you with the costs and headache of relocating.

Leasing Doctor Profile:
1. Someone who is unfamiliar or disinterested in maintenance
2. Someone who is not looking to grow the practice into a larger space
3. Someone who does not have the capital/ability to purchase a building outright

Owning Considerations:
1. Provides complete control over your destiny, building maintenance, aesthetics, signage (within local ordinances), etc.
2. Allows the dentist to passively build wealth (equity) by paying down the mortgage – at time for sale, you have an additional asset which can either be leased or sold.
3. Can be trickier to gain bank financing as a Commercial Real Estate (CRE) financing is likely going to be a separate loan from your practice. The bank may also require that you put capital down (i.e. – down payment) as CRE can be a riskier asset for a bank than a practice loan.
    Quick Tip – in the negotiation process (See Chapter 6) - consider having the seller carry the mortgage note (i.e. – seller financing).

Owning Doctor Profile:
1. Someone not afraid to take risks (above and beyond owning a practice)
2. Someone who is comfortable taking on additional maintenance tasks, or has a close friend/relative who can assist or provide advice on maintenance
3. Someone who is certain they will be practicing in THIS location for a reasonably long time
4. Someone who is wanting to complete a large-scale renovation to a building and/or its fixtures

Commercial Real Estate

In writing this book, I looked at other books on the market and noticed that many had the format and structure similar to a giant glossary of business terms. My endeavor has been to present the data in a more conversational tone and logical process. That said, I am about to make an exception and simply hit you with a few definitions. Commercial Real Estate is a unique industry where 'insiders' do often speak their own language of miscellaneous acronyms.

Here are a few of the key terms to learn:

CAM (Common Area Maintenance): This is an 'up' charge on your monthly rent rate, based on the landlord's costs to maintain the larger facility (snow plowing, landscaping, etc.). This is usually found when looking to rent a building in a multi-tenant facility (i.e. – strip-center or larger office building).

Base Term: This is the initial term in your lease (usually 5 or 10 years). After which, you should negotiate to have several options (usually 2-3) which provide you the right (but not requirement) to renew your contract for an additional amount of time (usually 5 years) for a pre-determined amount. Obviously, all of this is negotiable, even the rental rate when the term comes due.

TI (Tenant Improvements): TI is usually applicable to when you are building out or moving your location. Basically, it says that since the tenant (you) is willing to sign a longer-term contract (or if the landlord is having trouble leasing the space) they are willing to offset some of your costs of leasing a space by providing you money for construction / retrofitting. This can also be a tool used in negotiations as, most of you, are likely to be buying an older practice from a dentist who is retiring, as these practices usually are need of some updating. Obviously, you must be renting the space from someone who either has a cash base to support this or is a sophisticated commercial investor.

Lease Agreements: This is more of a general comment, that in your lease negotiations do ensure you have an attorney who is familiar with CRE. There are lots of different clauses which can come into play in your final lease agreement, you need legal representation who is very familiar with this type of negotiating / documentation. Read the lease carefully and highlight everything you do not understand for discussion with your lawyer. Remember, it is the lawyer's job to make sure you're signing a good piece of paper, it is your job to execute everything on that piece of paper.

How Much Will It Cost Me?

I have been looking forward to writing about this for some time, as I was taken off-guard by several costs that went into the practice purchase process. My goal is for you to have a full understanding of what you're going to be liable for in the month's leading up to your close date.

Bankers like to tell prospective clients that you need 'no money down' to get a practice loan. While this may be technically true (in the sense of a down payment), what they are not telling you is that there is still a significant invested required for the transaction to take place. Unfortunately, you will need to front a sizable amount of money in the months leading up to and immediately preceding your taking ownership.

Be thoughtful in planning your financials here. Make sure you have adequate cash reserves to afford this investment. Please do not attempt to buy a practice when you have no income after residency when you have $500 to your name. These costs are real, they add up quick and will absolutely need to be budgeted. While you can always delay purchases, hire a cheap attorney, avoid hiring an accountant, etc. – I would not recommend starting off my 20-30-year career cutting-corners. This is the time to be bold and take a leap of faith. Also keep in mind the words of Dr. Marvin Cohen (my wife's mentor) who always told her that 'cheap people pay twice'.

Below is a list of expenses I created using my wife's experience, along with some industry knowledge. PLEASE NOTE – that costs will vary by area, needs, and certainly personal preferences during the negotiation process. I included these only to give you some general guidance of how much money to have sitting on the sidelines, before pursuing a practice. Further, this list is not all-inclusive as costs will differ by practice and situation.

Possible Up-Front Expenses:
- Building Inspection: $750 - $1,000
- ALTA Land Survey: $2,000 - $3,000 (consider if buying)
- Building Appraisal: $2,000 - $3,000 (consider if buying)
- Title Insurance / Search: $250 - $750
- Lending Fee: $500 - $1,000
- Malpractice Insurance (1st Payment): $100 - $250
- Dental License: $250 - $500
- Initial Dental Equipment: $3,000 - $5,000
- Legal: $5,000 - $10,000
- Accounting: $3,000 - $5,000
- New Signage: $3,000 - $5,000
- Miscellaneous: $500 - $1,000
- **TOTAL: $20,350 - $35,750**

Do remember, that not everything listed above is required for your particular situation. For example, my wife did purchase her building, however we skipped the ALTA Land Survey and Appraisal (not always advisable, check with your attorney). While there was risk in doing so, it was a calculated risk that we felt comfortable with, given our situation at the time. Further, some of these costs may be able to be delayed until you are owning/operating the practice, making the 'out-of-pocket' costs much more bearable.

Quick Tip – Make sure you are tracking any money you spend on the practice search, negotiations, and closing process as this will all be tax deductible once you get your business up-and-running. This should include deductions for your mileage (driving to meet advisors, tour practices, etc.). Check with your accountant, of course, but since this is being done on behalf of 'the business' you should be able to claim it. I have included a worksheet to help you with tracking these expenses on FirstTimeDentist.com.

Creating You Practice Profile

Prior to sending out your first communication to any brokers, you may want to fill-out the following form as a way of helping guide the conversation on the type of practice in which you're trying to locate. Further, this will serve as a tool to 'keep you honest' throughout the process. The broker may find a screaming deal on a $3mm / year practice, but if you do not know how to run a team of 20, it is not much use to you.

Practice Profile Worksheet (available at FirstTimeDentist.com as well)

Specific Area Desired: _____

Prefer to: ☐ Own ☐ Lease

Interest in "Fixer-Upper" Practice? ☐ Yes, Please ☐ Never ☐ I'm Open

Looking for a Price Range of: $_____ - $_____

Looking for a Production Range of: $_____ - $_____

Looking for: ☐ Group Practice ☐ Solo Practice ☐ Associateship

CAD/CAM: ☐ Required ☑ Not Required

Business Model: ☐ Bread & Butter' ☐ Underserved ☐ Aesthetic
☐ Family ☐ Mixed ☐ Other_____

Desired Number of Days Worked / Week: _____

Desired Number of Employees: _____

Desired Number of Operatories: _____

Background on yourself:

Where do you go to school? Why did you become a dentist? Why do you want to practice in this area? Discuss your family, your interests, etc. Give them a taste of WHO you are and WHY you want to buy a practice. Remember – many of these individuals have owned their practices for years. Their patients are close friends. Their employees may be almost family members – they want to know that whomever they are selling to is someone that has earned the right long-term fit.

Practice Search Tactics

There are several approaches to practice searches that you may employ, depending on your area and site availability. Outside of doing a basic online search for practices for sale in XX area, there are several other more creative ways to go about your search. Below, I put together a list of ideas to assist you in making contacts and developing some practice leads.

Remember – this is hand-to-hand combat, you need to be looking for referrals, recommendations, and people who know people. There is no Zillow.com[xix] or mass data collector for available dental practices. Even if there were, some of the best practices / deals may be ones that are not yet on the market.

Individuals / Organizations to Contact:
1. Dental Practice Brokers - Most straight-forward search, goes straight to the source. The issue is that you're only going to see listings for each broker (unless you hire one to represent you).
2. Nearest Dental School - Dental schools have large amounts of staff members who have been in the dental field for a while. Someone there may know of a friend or colleague who is looking to transition.
3. Chamber of Commerce - The Local Chamber of Commerce is likely a repository of non-public information about who is business is doing well, who wants to retire/sell, etc. Even if they do not give you a direct lead, they may help you make contact with individuals who have 'connections'.
4. Dental Specialists - Do an online search for all the Ortho's, Endo's, Pedo's Perio's, Oral Surgeons, etc. and see if they have any referring doctors who they would recommend to contact. They work with General Dentists daily and likely have an inside scoop.
5. Dental Suppliers - Suppliers have a unique insight into dental practices as they work closely with their clients on a daily or weekly basis. Additionally, they usually cover a broad, but specific geographic area. These individuals are likely connected with the local 'gossip' as well, which is critical for finding those hidden gems of future practices for sale.
6. Dental Societies - Many areas have local dental meetings one a monthly or quarterly basis. Try contacting the head of this group for a meeting schedule or any inside-information they can provide.
7. Financial Advisors / Accountants - Use your own advisors or seek out other advisors, they likely would need their client's permission to share your information, but this could foster some results.
8. Mass broadcast – post in a larger forum or dental magazine, it can be a bit of a shot-in-the-dark, but it is free, easy and can reach quite a few people (who usually know equally as many people).
9. Cold-Calling – Individually contact each dental practice in your target area. Consider using [ESRI's Business Analyst Online](#) free trial to find your target market and all the dentists working in that market.

This can be one of the dicer approaches as it requires all the stars to align in your unique situation, as well as the doctors on the receiving end. That said, it is the most assertive approach to finding a practice. Do be selective, however. Do not mail everyone, get a list – drive the offices, call the front desks, and read online reviews before contacting.

As with any of these scenarios, make sure you use some discretion. Depending on your situation, you may not want to broadcast that fact that you're looking to buy a practice (i.e. – if you're trying to get out of an associateship).

If this is the case, do not be afraid to use your lawyer, accountant, etc. to be your 'face' in the search process. For example, you could have the lawyer send out a letter you create (on their letterhead) which states that 'their client' is searching for a certain type of dental practice. This allows your advisor's name to be attached to the request and then they can forward any responses directly to you.

Recap

After completing this chapter, I hope that you have a deep understanding of how to start your search and what you want out of a practice.

Searching for your practice is one of the biggest unknowns in terms of timing, for the entire practice purchase process. I can probably estimate within a tolerance of a few days / week of how long most steps will take. This step, however, is very individualized and specific to your needs, wants, desired area, acceptable risk, practice availability, etc.

To get to the punchline – this part of the process could last longer than expected and cause you quite a bit of frustration ('I just can't find what I'm looking for...'). My advice is to be determined and keep your focus on the vision you set out to accomplish. You need to treat finding a practice like a game, one which your unwilling to forfeit or fail. If there's one thing I've learned in working in the commercial real estate industry, it is that real estate always 'turns-over'. Somehow, someway a space always comes available. It may not occur when you want, but it will come available if you are patient enough.

Please take this sage advice and attitude with you into your practice search. Stay patient that something will turnover, confident in your decisions to search, and whatever you do – do not settle for something just because of availably. Wait-it-out to get exactly what you want.

CHAPTER 4: PRELIMINARY DUE DILIGENCE

"Not deciding, is the coward's way of quitting. If you're going to quit – do not let it come from inactivity. Quit, only after you have failed gloriously..." -- Dream Year (Ben Arment)

We're finally at the point where we can start analyzing your potential practice and coming up with a plan on which practices to pursue. Think about this process like you would searching for your first home. You've decided on what type of house you want, generally, where you want to live, and how many kids you may or may not have in the future. You've created a vision and set the parameters on what is acceptable, now it is time to execute.

From here, in the house hunting process, you would probably begin to review housing 'leads' online from sites and start looking at pictures, mortgage, and neighborhoods to see if the house is worth visiting or not.

The dental practice process is similar in this regard, in that you want to begin assembling a small group of practices that are within a certain distance of your target market. You can then begin to categorize them and/or remove them from your consideration set.

The first two steps I would recommend taking are seeing the practice location in person and then performing a mystery shop of the practice. I would suggest doing these *prior* to making known your formal interest with a broker or signing an Non-Disclosure Agreement. In this case, anonymity can be one of your most powerful assets when reviewing the less tangible characteristics of a practice.

Beyond surveying the location and mystery shopping, I'm going to present you with some basic metrics and data to consider when assessing practices for sale. Use this information to 'weed out' the practices that are an unlikely fit for your vision. Remember, you put together the vision for a reason – if you find a really attractive practice that focuses on high-end dentistry, but you only want to do 'bread-and-butter' dentistry – do not try to convince yourself that you can make it work. Either the practice is aligned with your vision, or it is not. If it is not, you can still conceptualize the process and possibility of converting it to your vision, over time. Just know that this type of cultural shift can be a long road with the existing employees and patients (5-10 years).

Location Analysis

People use the phrase "Location, Location, Location" quite often. The truth is, that phrase is missing a key component and that's a fourth 'Location'! Objectively analyzing the exterior look/feel, the accessibility, and the neighborhood demographics of a potential practice are important. Outside of the patient demographic, having the location in alignment with your vision is one of the most important things you can do for your future success.

In my years working as a strategist in the location analytics, we spent copious amounts of time pouring over the most minute details of a potential branch location. We would look at things like traffic lights, speed limits, signage, if the site was above/below grade, competitor locations/signage, building size/prominence, future traffic pattern changes, nearby businesses, type / quality of neighborhoods, and a host of demographic statistics.

My point is that the significant amount of time we spent looking at a potential location, was directly correlated with the fact that we were spending upwards of $3 Million (or more) to acquire, construct, and open a new bank branch. While you spend is hopefully a fraction of this, it is still likely to be the single biggest purchase of your life. Thus, spending some time analyzing the details could pay off in the long-run.

I would recommend visiting the practice during regular business hours so that you can get an idea as to the level of foot/vehicle traffic, as well as the patient demographic. I know this may seem a bit strange, but I would try to plan on an hour to visit the practice, fill out the assessment and perhaps even just sit and observe or canvas the nearby area. Even if you are familiar with the location or area, it will be time well spent as you will be surprised at the amount of unforeseen qualities that you will get to observe. For example, my colleagues and I believe that we once witnessed a drug deal in the parking lot of a prospective location we were analyzing – had we not been literally sitting there observing, we would not have noticed. It certainly made us think differently about pursuing that site!

Below is a list of site evaluation criteria. So, plan out your incognito trip and whether you camp-out in your car, at a nearby bench and just observe and take notes.

What Type of Location is the Prospective Practice?:

1. Free-Standing Building
2. In-Line (Strip Center)
3. Office Building
4. Other

<u>Importance</u>: usually a Free-Standing building offers greater level of visibility, which helps support your brand in the community, as well as make it easier for people to find the building for the first time. That said, look at the competitors in the area – would you out-position them with a bigger/more attractive building? That said, Free-Standing are usually the costliest and may require that you own vs. lease.

It is also worth mentioning that in some markets (i.e. – densely populated/urban areas) the only real estate you may be able to find is In-Line or Office Building, this is why understanding your market and competitors is very important. In these cases, it is likely more important to note what floor you are on, the type of signage that's available, or the proximity to public transportation or downtown work centers.

Visibility: _____ (report card scale: A-F)

<u>What to look for</u>: Drive past the location and/or walk around it. How far away can you see the location? Are there trees or landscaping that will impede visibility in the spring/summer months? Are there buildings being built nearby or is there room for future construction? This could impede your visibility.

Accessibility: _____ (report card scale: A-F)

<u>What to look for</u>: How easy is it to find and access the practice? Are you on a 25-mph street or 50 (faster speeds make it more difficult to identify and slow down)? Are there stop signs, traffic signals, or medians which impede access? Do they need to cross the street? If you're in an urban area – where are the nearest stops for public

One quick recommendation, call the local planning department to see if there are any planned projects or road construction. I once read about an individual who bought a practice only to find that major road construction commenced after they closed. Issues with traffic patterns can cause additional patient cancellations or cause them to be late and back up your schedule. Simply call your local planning/permits office and tell them that you are considering purchasing a building on XX street and wanted to know if there are any planned projects in the near future.

Parking / Mass Transit :
On-Site parking? _____ **(Y/N)**
Distance to Mass Transit_____ **(Miles/Minutes)**

<u>What to look for</u>: The parking situation can be extremely important to ensure the best possible experience for new patients. If there is not On-Site parking (ideal), where are customers expected to park? How far of a walk is it? If it is paid, will you be validating parking? In terms of parking spots, I would recommend a minimum of 1 parking spot per operatory to cover the spaces needed for patients, not employees. Do you have/need employee parking? Do you need to pay for their parking?

If you are in a more dense / urban area – how accessible is public transportation? Where is the nearest train stop, bus stop or otherwise to the prospective practice? Is it a primary transit line or more of a secondary line? How 'walkable' is the nearby area?

Signage: _____ **(report card scale: A-F)**

<u>What to look for</u>: What type of sign does the current doctor have? Is it new or old? What do the newest signs in the area look like (may inform you of what you're likely to get, given local code). Is it free-standing, or attached to the building? Is it a panel on a larger sign for a retail center? How big is the sign in comparison to other businesses in the area? Do any of the signs have lighting?

You may want to comb through the community's planning department website to see if there are posted regulations on the amount, type, and size of permitted signage. This could also be worth a call to the planning department to see if there have been signage code updates or 'overlays', as these would affect all new / nongrandfathered signage. Point is, do not necessarily assume that you can get the same signage as the seller.

Nearby Businesses:

<u>What to look for</u>: You also want to look at your neighboring retailers. In the commercial real estate business, there is something called 'gravity theory' why retail centers are typically large clusters of businesses in a small geographic area vs. being dispersed over larger areas.

Neighborhood Notes:

<u>What to look for</u>: Spend some time taking in your surroundings. Are there lots of vacant retailers/for lease signs? Broken windows or vandalism? Is there a new development being built? New homes? What type of housing is nearby (single/multi-family)? How big are the homes/apartment units? Are the public utilities and infrastructure intact and functional? What type of cars are driving past you? This section is pretty open-ended but write down anything interesting you see about the neighborhood or the demographic frequenting the area.

Remember, if you want to practice high-end dentistry, but are considering a location down the street from some seedy retail stores – you're likely to end up with a lot of people walking in who are not your target audience. However, if you want to do family dentistry, positioning yourself next to a grocery store can be a convenient way for parents to drop off kids for a cleaning and then run next store to pick-up milk.

Use this questionnaire as a way of being honest with yourself about what your potential practice has to offer. Judge everything on the basis of what you would ideally want. I know that I keep coming back to your 'vision', but it is crucial that you make sure that this potential is fully aligned with your needs/desires. Exercise caution in continuing the process if you are trying to rationalize pursing this particular practice.

If, however, you come back to the data you collected in a day or so and find that you still have a strong interest in the practice, I would heavily recommend getting up-close and personal with the practice through a Mystery Shop.

FIRST TIME DENTIST

Mystery Shopping

Before you start the process of identifying yourself and making data requests, it may behoove you to plan a 'Mystery Shop' of all possible dental practices. Mystery Shopping involves going into a particular business (companies will actually hire people to do this) and walk through the normal course of a transaction / interaction with their employees. It is a way of gaining clean objective view on the qualitative factors.

Once you identify yourself, the doctor and staff (if they know) will certainly treat you differently than if you were the average Joe patient walking in off the street. If you are unable to mystery shop the location in person, consider hiring a friend or family member to help. Take them out to a nice dinner and discuss their findings. You could be present with them when they setup their initial appointment and listen to the phone conversation or (even better) setup the appointment for them – you get the interaction and they do not have to do it. Creativity may be required to procure this 'soft' but crucial information in your decision process.

Regardless of your approach, below is a list of steps I would recommend taking for an in-person mystery shop, along with associated questions and observations that you should document. This type of qualitative information is incredible, both from a purchase perspective and from a future management perspective. This is your one and only chance for you, the doctor, to gain first-hand, objective information about this practice. Once you sign the Non-Disclosure Agreement, meet doctor and (hopefully) become the owner – you will never again have this opportunity.

I know it may seem awkward at first, but the more you turn this into a game, the better your result. See how far you can push and probe the staff and doctor by asking some 'borderline' questions on how the office runs or on any other topic that comes to mind during your visit.

Unfortunately for my wife, she was unable to perform a mystery shop as she had somewhat of an inside scoop on her practice. My mother-in-law was, in fact, a substitute hygienist at her practice for several years prior to my wife's purchase. While my wife was unable to gain the first-hand knowledge of the inner workings of, what would someday be her practice – she was still able to slyly ask her mom questions about operations or staff - without her knowing the intent, which did prove to be valuable in the end.

In our case, the tricky part was the fact that up until a few weeks beforehand, my mother-in-law did _not_ know we were looking into buying the practice. In fact, we had kept it a secret from both of our families for quite some time up until this point. More on this topic in our next chapter, however.

The reason I bring this up is due to the sage insights my mother-in-law has always brought about, regarding her experiences as an RDH. One of her recurring comments goes something like the following, when prefacing a unique story about an anonymous patient:

"...I swear, as I soon as I lay them back in their chair, it is like their arms cross and the floodgates open. Sometimes I'm convinced that they mistake me for a psychiatrist as they will spill their entire life stories".

Why is this important? Hygienists spend a lot of time with patients. The time can be very personal and somewhat intimate (I mean, they are digging around in your mouth for heaven-sakes!). It is not unusual for Hygienists to have a special connection with patients which may supersede that of the doctor's. They both listen to things patients amazingly forget to tell the dentist 10 minutes later, as well as <u>tell</u> the patients things about the office or dentist.

Point is, you're likely to get the most in-depth and authentic view of the practice, while you are physically in the practice (probably laying on your back staring at the ceiling tiles). Thus, do not take any conversation with any staff member for granted, make good use of your time in the practice and please take copious notes when you're finished!

As with everything in this exercise, you'll want to test the entire process 'end-to-end'. Start by finding an advertisement, web-site, or some other means of contacting the office.

First Contact:
1. Is their contact information easy to find?
2. What did the website look like? Was it easy to navigate for new patients?
3. Do they offer on-line appointment booking? Are the hours convenient?
4. Next, you will want to call and make a prophy appointment. Take note of all the interactions that you have with their front desk.

Making the Appointment:
1. Did they answer by the second ring? Or did you go to voicemail?
2. If you went to voicemail – how long before they called back?
3. Was the person you spoke with friendly? Knowledgeable (not fumbling around trying to make appointment)?
4. Were you put on hold? How long?
5. How long do you have to wait to get an appointment?
6. Did they ask you about your medical history? Why you needed a new dentist? Or any other qualitative assessment into your background?

Remember as you go through this exercise, every item listed above can be changed once you take over. You can/will have a new website, advertising, you can train new front desk interactions and protocol. The key is that you are building the story for this practice. You are trying to understand the establishment in which these patients are used to interacting. You want to see and feel everything from the patient's point of view, while you have the opportunity to do so in an unbiased manner.

Develop Your Story:
Before you leave for your first appointment, spend a few minutes developing a persona – remember you may need to tell a few white lies or stretch the truth as you are trying to get the most honest experience possible

Are you new to town (always a good one)? What type of work do you do (but do not tell them you are a dentist)? Do you have a family? How long have you lived in the area? Perhaps your mom used to be a dental hygienist (hence your clean teeth)? Uncle is a dentist and moved to another state? Just make sure you have one layer's worth of information below these items. If your mom is a hygienist, it is possible that the someone would ask 'where' and 'for whom' do they work?

Remember, the goal is not to go in with a completely different name, hairdo, and make up lies about your personal life – but having a few answers to common pleasantry questions is good preparation

The First Impression:
This is when it gets exciting, as you begin to pull into your parking spot at the dental office. Your blood pressure starts to rise a bit as you begin to think of the possibility of it being your name on the side of the building, not someone else's. You may have some initial butterflies as it looks like the perfect practice you have dreamed of, or you are crushed because the building is ugly, it is in a bad part of town, or its simply not what you expected.

All these feelings are inevitable, but this is not the time for emotion. Think of yourself like a special forces unit in the military, they show up to perform a mission and they are not thinking of all that could or should be in regards to their situation. Their focus – the mission. Save the emotion for closing day and the rest of your career. Doing so will also help you to avoid talking yourself into our out of the practice too early. At this point, you may not even know what the finances look like.

For now, we're also not going to focus too much on the exterior experience of the building, as that is covered later in this chapter ("Location Analysis"). The thing to focus on here is what does it feel like, from a patient's perspective, to walk in through the front doors and have your first interaction with the office staff. Do go into this appointment 15-20 minutes early, remember as you're sitting in the waiting room, you can be on your phone stealthy taking notes (see the Evernote[xx] app).

Here are some questions to ask yourself why you are waiting:
1. What is the first word that comes to mind as you walk through the front door?
2. Does the office strike you as clean, updated, lots of natural light? Or is the office dirty, old, or dark?
3. Does the office and furniture appear to be clean?
4. Are there magazines, free WIFI, a TV or other waiting room entertainment?

Quick Tip – Look at the age on the magazines – are they all less than 3 or so months old? If they are a year old, it tells you that the office may lack some systems as no one is keeping these fresh.

5. Does the doctor have any self-promotion ("ask us about...") or educational information in the waiting room?
6. Are there 'sticky' notes or cheesy clip art signs to the patients?
7. What is the demographic of the other patients in the waiting room?
8. Are you immediately greeted? Does the front desk look happy and welcoming?
9. Is the front desk / back office clean or disorganized and chaotic?

Obviously, first impressions are key in most anything in life. Think of your spouse or significant other. While you may not have said "I am going to marry this person" the first time you met them, it is very unlikely that you thought to yourself "there is no way I could marry this person" when you first met them.

The Staff:
Make sure you covertly watch the staff's every move. You're trying to observe how they interact with other patients, with other staff members, and the dentist. Listen intently to the language they use, how they use it, and how they manage patient flow. Try to eavesdrop on neighboring conversations and activity throughout the office.

Here are some questions to consider:

1. Does the staff gather or appear to be gossiping anywhere in the office?
2. Is anyone using their cellphone and/or texting?
3. Are they friendly or rude? Helpful or not concerned with you?
4. Do they appear put together? Clean scrubs? Professional looking?
5. Does the hygienist follow all sterilization or other compliance protocols (best you can tell)?
6. Do they discuss any dental/clinical topics or only personal?

The Prophy:

As I mentioned in the earlier part of this chapter, the conversations you will have with the staff are key. The conversation you will have with the hygienist is probably one of the most important and intimate discussions that will take place. However, you will not want to forget about the more technical side of dental hygiene as you're going through the appointment.

Questions to consider:
1. When your name is called in the waiting room and you begin walking back to the exam room, is there a staff member walking beside you or in-front of you? Or did they 'run-off' to the room after your name was verbalized?
2. Does anyone provide a brief tour of the office? Perhaps showcasing a new piece of technology (neat looking digital pan, CAD/CAM unit, etc.)?
3. What is your first impression of the layout of the office?
4. What is your first impression of the exam rooms? Are there chairs clean and updated or tattered and old?
5. What questions do they ask you when you are seated? Standard stuff (hopefully / at a minimum)? Anything outside the ordinary?
6. Does the hygienist ask any more probing questions on your past dental experiences, concerns with oral health, etc.? Or do they tell you about their kid's soccer game the entire time?
7. Does the hygienist strike a balance between talking about their personal life, your personal life and dental education?
8. Did the hygienist appear to have all the necessary equipment in the exam room or did they have to leave mid-appointment for anything?

Remember, now is the time to ask the hygienist some questions about the office. Do not be afraid to push the bounds a bit...

9. How long have you worked here?
10. Might lead into another question like how they like current practice vs. old practice (if they are newer to the office)?
11. Or, if the person has been there a while ask why they like the practice so much?
12. How long has Dr. X owned the practice?
13. Ask how busy they are, how many days a week they are open, if they work a certain time on a certain day, etc.
14. How many patients does the practice have? How many do you see each day?

The questions should all be general and open-ended. You are trying to open up a conversation of them saying something like "Yes we're working 6 days a week and do not have room for patients" or "About a year ago business started to slow so we've been cutting back days". Remember, you do not want to pepper the hygienist with questions, this is more so a list of ideas to strike up a deeper conversation.

The Dentist:

In terms of the mystery shop of the dentist is probably the second most important portion of your visit (behind the hygiene appointment). You want to understand, in this brief encounter, how the dentist manages their patient interaction. If you can, while waiting for them to enter, try to eavesdrop on neighboring conversations the dentist may be having with patients.

<u>Some questions to consider:</u>

1. Did the dentist come in on time? If not, did they apologize? Were they sincere?
2. What is your first impression of the dentist? How does the dentist greet you?
3. Does the dentist look professional? Is he/she dressed in scrubs or more formal attire?
4. Does he/she attempt to get to know you? Or are they in a hurry?
5. How does the dentist treat the staff? Kindly? Or more of a dictator?
6. Would you want this dentist working on your grandmother?
7. Did the dentist diagnose or prescribe any type of treatment? Do you agree with the treatment plan?
8. Does the dentist and/or hygienist give you clear instructions on when you can leave and where the check-out desk is located?
9. Does the dentist shake your hand before leaving?
10. If you were a patient, would you want to come back to this dentist?

Check-Out:

Lastly, we need to make sure that you are properly escorted from the dental exam chair out to the front desk and out of the office in clean flowing manner.

<u>Questions to consider:</u>
1. Did someone walk you up to the front desk or were you given directions?
2. How long did you have to wait at the front desk to be acknowledged?
3. Did the front desk reschedule you for your next cleaning or other appointment?
4. Were they courteous on your way out? Thank you for coming in?
5. Did they ask if you have any family or friends that need appointments?
6. Were you given / offered appointment reminder cards?

When you're finished with your visit, make sure you write down everything you learned into a notebook or type it up. In fact, do not even leave the office yet. Go into your car or find a quiet place nearby that you can sit down and recount/document your experience. This is great information for you to refer back to, later in the process.

As I will go on to say several times, there are very few true 'deal-breakers' in this process – especially when it comes to qualitative data. The point here is that you have a unique opportunity to take a view of the office that you will never again be allotted. Spend the time and money!

Non-Disclosure Agreement

Now that you had the opportunity to collect some anonymous data, you will need to make a 'Go/No-Go' decision on whether or not to pursue this particular practice. Hopefully the practice is aligned with your vision and you want to start analyzing the numbers. To do so, you will need to get in contact with the broker and simply let them know that you are interested in learning more.

Prior to getting 'under the hood' on your first practice, a practice broker will probably request that you sign a non-disclosure agreement or NDA. An NDA is something to be taken very seriously as it is intended to protect the business interests of the seller.

Why is an NDA required? Basically what the seller is trying to avoid adverse impacts to his business, as a way of preserving the most valuable asset in a practice (Goodwill[xxi]).

For example, the seller is trying to avoid a scenario in which you tell the entire dental community that the practice is for sale, the patients (or employees) find out and get nervous about the change and start going to other dentists. The subsequent loss of patients (and goodwill) could lead to a reduced price for the seller. Remember – the majority of what you will be buying is the practice's goodwill, not the fixed assets (equipment, building, inventory, furniture, etc.).

The NDA could cover many different aspects in terms of timing, who can be involved on your side for the transaction, etc. There are lots of situations that may be covered in an NDA, the only advice I would have is to make sure that there are no restrictions on the sharing of data with your own representatives. Any and all information you are privy to should be shared with all of your team, in order to achieve the best outcome. Review this document thoroughly before signing, and chat with your lawyer if you have questions!

For my wife and I, this was one of the more challenging portions of the due diligence process. For us, we were both living in separate parts of the state and had begun to think about the idea of moving back to my wife's hometown in Southern Ohio. Doing so, would have immediately set off red flags to some in and around the dental community.

First off, remember that my mother-in-law was involved in the community since she subbed at the office. Considering the fact that she worked for a dentist who was nearing the end of his career, it is not rocket science to put two-and-two together that Dr. Heim is moving home (to a small town), her mom works here, current dentist is retirement age, and she is also going to be a dentist...hmm.

Retrospect, we did probably make this into a bigger deal than it needed to be, however at the time it created quite a bit of stress. We were moving to a smaller town and could not afford to buy a home so we needed to rent. I found that it is very difficult to find a rental home in a small town (where rental search engines are less effective), especially when you live 2-4 hours away.

Eventually we gained special approval from the selling doctor to give us the ability to discuss this with our families. This gave us some peace of mind as we were then able to ask for help (from her family) in locating a rental home. Doing so also alleviated some stress as we had these impending dates (our wedding / wife finishing residency) and people kept incessantly asking us 'what' we would be doing afterwards. Given that this is a pretty logical question, it is very hard to skirt the answer for too long. Further, while it is fairly easy to avoid the topic and/or tell white lies to friends and acquaintances, it is much harder to do the same to your parents with whom you hopefully have a much deeper and trustful relationship.

When I look back now, I do laugh about this 'secret' we were keeping and for how long we kept it. However, there is good reason for keeping things secret, as we already discussed. Do not underestimate the power of a legal contract. As my own lawyer quoted when we were signing our NDA... 'loose lips sink ships.'

Preliminary Data Request

Immediately after signing the NDA, you have officially entered the due diligence[xxii] phase. The broker should provide you with a host of information, below are a few things that should be included, if the broker does not deliver any or all of this information, I would not hesitate to go back and ask for it to be sent over. DO NOT EVER feel reluctant to ask for more data or clarification, when needed. Due diligence is a process built to support the potential buyer in evaluating and determining the best course of action.

While the seller has the right to ensure you are a good 'match' for his/her practice, the onus is on you to request and analyze all appropriate information.

Data Request Checklist:
1. **Practice Overview Packet**: summary level information that broker assembles, not necessary but a helpful way of condensing information
2. **Tax Returns**: minimum of three years of federal tax returns
3. **Production Schedule**: 1 years' worth of doctor and hygiene production by dental code
4. **Staffing Survey**: List of all employees, length of employment, position, pay, benefits, full-time/part-time, vacation days and rating (A-F) on performance. Job descriptions, if available, would also be helpful. (See FirstTimeDentist.com for example survey).
5. **Building and/or Practice Appraisals**: the latter may be open to interpretation if the seller's broker completed the appraisal (if owned)
6. **Fee Schedules**: Get the list of all the PPOs the seller participates with, along with their associated fee schedules (some PPOs have different 'levels' make sure that's included) as well as the seller's fee schedule.
7. **Practice Financials**: three years' worth of the P&L (profit and loss) income statement. This will help you understand how the practice's overhead
8. **Accounts Receivable**: total amount of outstanding balances due to the practice.
9. **Credit Balances**: total amount of balances the practice owes to patients (overpaid accounts), this amount will be subtracted from the Accounts Receivable when you purchase the practice.
10. **Building Layout**: ideally, a floorplan showing how location is 'setup', walls, offices, operatories, etc. (in case you didn't mystery shop)
11. **Equipment List**: detailed list of all dental equipment, including equipment type, brand, when purchased, etc. – can also be completed for each operatory
12. **Patient Counts**: Number of active patients (seen in last 18 months)
13. **Employee Manual**: If available, get a copy of the employee manual
14. **Miscellaneous Facts**: Number of new patients / month, hours open, vacation days provided, continuing education policy, employee dental benefits, etc.

Throughout the remainder of the book, we will utilize data points from these reports for further analysis and review. For now, just make sure that you have each of these items and immediately request anything that is missing. As you will find, sometimes the 'turn-around time' of making a data request can be lengthy, even for a simple item.

Keep in mind that you are typically making the request to the broker, the broker making the request to the seller, and potentially the seller asking an employee to pull the data, and then getting it back to you. The point is that sometimes it can take a few days to get information returned to you, so make you're requests early so that you're not waiting on crucial information later in the process.

Practice Financials

In the finance and accounting industry, there are two types of accounting that exist: Financial and Managerial[xxiii]. Think of "Financial" as you would Wall-Street, the IRS, the SEC, or other major government regulators. While Managerial reporting is a set of internal reports which help managers run the business day-to-day.

In dentistry, there is a similar distinction to make in that we report-out a certain type of financials to the IRS each year (i.e. – financial reporting). These are typically generated through QuickBooks or a similar accounting software and either maintained by or thoroughly checked by your accountant.

While I will touch on parts of financial accounting throughout this document and my web-site, I would by-and-large default to discussing these types of financials with your accountant. Your accountant will be able to dig-through 3 years of the practice's tax returns (standard request) and properly adjust / interpret them to give you the best view of financial performance.

However, where I will spend a majority of my time trying to help you understand the other end of the spectrum – Managerial Financials. The following are list of key metrics, along with industry benchmarks and a description on each metric. Reviewing these metrics in print can be somewhat tedious, so I have put together a workbook on FirstTimeDentist.com which should help you quickly evaluate your prospective practice. This workbook allows you to entire a short list of data points and analyze an easy set of graphs and charts.

Year-over-Year (YoY) Growth

Since prices are always increasing (cost of supplies, wages, equipment, utilities, etc.) we need to ensure that a practice is growing it is 'top-line' production YoY.

<u>Negative or flat growth (<0% to 2%)</u> – could suggest the doctor has cut hours, insurance, marketing or otherwise. At some point this becomes unsustainable, so you need to understand the factors at play and decide whether you can reverse them. If the underlying factor is a loss of jobs and decline in the economy, it is going to be tough to improve that organically.

<u>Moderate Growth (2% to 5%)</u> – likely where most practices are at, when a doctor is nearing retirement. They are not looking to greatly expand, just steady growth.

<u>Strong Growth (5% to 15%)</u> – Growth above 5% is certainly desirable, but you should also begin to look at the doctor's formula. Why have they been able to sustain constant / strong growth? Did they hire a strong marketing agency? Diligence on fee increases each year?

<u>Significant Growth (15%+)</u> – similar to the negative or flat growth, a strong growth trend can be difficult to sustain. Just from a staffing / building capacity perspective, adding 15% a year in production (unless solely through fees, which would eventually reduce your competitiveness) is likely to cause you strain. How much more can you grow in your current space with your current team? Can you build on or expand the space? Do you want to do that? What are the underlying factors for growth, low profit margins due to high marketing expense? New associate? Etc.?

You should shoot for at least 5% annual average growth (remember this includes fee increases which should be done on a regular basis). However, if you see significant negatives or huge increases – these are things to ask the broker – not always a deal breaker - was there an illness in the family? Road construction? Did they hire/fire a temporary associate?

Collections Ratio

Collections are one of the most important metrics in your business, because it is the lifeblood, the cashflow that keeps the lights on and employees paid. As such, it is important to understand what percent of the office's total production is being 'taken home' (Total Collections / Total Production over a given time period). Depending on your business model (percent of production which is Fee-for-Service vs. PPO vs. Medicaid), you may see a large swing in the collection ratio. Regardless, here are a few rough guidelines to consider when looking at the office's collection ratio:

Best-in-Class: 98%+
Tolerable: 95-98%
Needs Improvement: <95%

Reasons why your Collections Ratio is less than 100%

1. Insurance: is probably one of the largest influencers on the collections ratio. The difference between your fee and fee schedule you have agreed to with a PPO is written-off (not collected). Attempting to collect monies above and beyond the agreed upon fee schedules will get you in a mess of legal trouble.

2. Voluntary Write-Offs: these occur when a patient has a bad experience, is planning on doing additional work (and you provide a discount), or just out of the kindness of your own heart. Regardless, you will want to monitor any write-offs which occur outside of insurance. Having a process in place which requires the Dr.'s approval is ideal.

Remember, regardless of whether or not you charge a patient for a procedure, you should always, always be booking them procedure in the system. The first reason you want to do this is to allow for there to be a coherent paper trail. You want documentation of what you did to each patient, even if you did not charge! Second, it is a good business practice – showing the patient that they otherwise would have been charged $300 for the procedure can leave them feeling good about their experience that day.

3. Fraud: While there are many forms of fraud and this is likely harder to detect in the practice purchase process, since you likely do not have full / daily access to the management software, I thought it was still worth mentioning. This is one of the areas where someone could be embezzling funds from the business, by taking payments from patients for procedures which are then written-off, thereby driving down the collections ratio.

4. Process: Depending on how the office systems are setup, it is possible that the money has been produced, the patients may even be willing to pay – the business has just not notified them that they owe the money yet! You often hear horror stories about single provider practices who, for lack of knowledge, motivation or understanding, are operating with $100k or more in accounts receivable. That's money in your pocket, all you have to do is go get it!

Accounts Receivable

When you purchase a practice, you will likely need to purchase the accounts receivable as well. This is basically the backlog of everyone who owes you money whether insurance companies or patients. We will discuss more about buying the accounts receivable in a later chapter. However, given the current topic of collections processes, I think it is important to understand how to interpret these metrics.

Figure 4.1: Sample AR Report:

<30 Days	30-60 Days	60-90 Days	>90 Days	Total
$57,000	$10,000	$5,000	$3,000	$75,000
76.0%	13.3%	6.7%	4%	100.0%

In the example above, the total AR is $75k. That means, that the Dr. has done $75k worth of dentistry for which they have not been paid. However, the good thing here is that nearly 90% of the balances are less than 60 days. Usually the < 30 days are simply in the process of being refunded (from insurance) or paid by the patients.

The 30-60-day bucket and 60-90 Day buckets should be your priority for whoever does the collections in your office. These are either patients who have fallen behind in paying or insurance companies disputing coverage/procedures. Each account in these buckets should have a 'story' attached to it, that your collections manager can explain. In that, there either waiting on the insurance company to reprocess with correct information, the patient is coming back for more work next week, or perhaps the patient had a family emergency and you're waiting to resend the bill. Whatever the story is, one needs to exist, otherwise it is not being actively worked.

The likelihood that you will collect funds goes down the 'older' the account becomes. As such, for the 90+ bucket, you mind as well consider the work done for these patients to have been a donation. You will likely achieve a single digit collection rate on any funds in this category. From a process perspective, if you find a great deal of accounts in this 90+ bucket, you should consider hiring a collections attorney. They can be fairly priced and if you consider the fact that the funds are unlikely to be collected by you. Even say that with lots of diligence and time you collect 10% of the 90+ AR bucket, you can compare that to collecting 33% of the funds and paying the attorney 33%, you would end up collecting 22% (vs. the 10%). Here is a quick example which shows you how you can calculate the expected AR collection rate

Why am I rambling on about AR management when you do not even own the business yet? First off, you will be buying the funds, so it is good to understand the quality of the accounts that you are buying. I think it is important to understand the state of the AR as it is likely a good indicator of the effectiveness of the business processes which are in place. It is quite easy to show up to work and just deal with 'putting out the fires' for that day. AR becomes something you will get around to in the afternoon, then the afternoon gets busy and you will handle it tomorrow. Next thing you know, you are one of the dentists with a good chunk of your annual salary sitting in 'limbo'.

If you see total accounts receivable that exceed of monthly production by a significant amount, you should consider further investigating the process (or lack thereof) the practice has for collections. Further, if you do find issues, you will want to consider a plan for how to immediately address those upon your taking over.

Accounts Receivable Turn Ratio:

The Turn ratio helps you understand how quickly you are 'turning' over AR balances into actual cash in your pocket. To calculate, simply take the Total AR / Average Monthly Production. What this ratio will tell you is the average time frame it takes for you to get your money.

For example, a $100k AR balance for a $50k / month production practice would say that it takes 2 months for you to get paid on your production. Ideally, you want to see this metric to be at or below 1, meaning you're collecting your money within 1 month (or even less). As we saw in the AR example above, the rate of collections goes down and employee time chasing insurance companies or patients goes up, as time progresses.

Overhead

Overhead is simply a measure of how much of your collections is being spent to support business activities (Total Expenses / Total Collections). Overhead is necessary and, quite honestly, too little overhead is not necessarily a good thing – as this can be a sign that the practice is not re-investing into itself.

In terms of overhead, there are many thoughts on what a 'good' ratio is – I think a lot of this is dependent on your local area / market competitiveness, here are a few quick rules of thumb:

High: 70-80%

Find out where the owner is spending the money, and why. Keep in mind the spending can be justifiable (new equipment, advanced training, consulting, etc.) – you just need to understand the reasons as they may not necessarily indicate a bad situation. If, however, you see the overhead is extremely high due to long-term employee salaries – this is a problem as you may have trouble continuing to pay them cause a host of downstream impacts.

Moderate: 60-70%
For the new dentist, this range is probably where you will start, as you will need to service debt, likely re-invest into the business (renovations, new equipment, etc.). Overhead in this range is more 'business as usual' – the owner is probably not overly investing in the business, but they are also not under-investing

Low: 50-60%
Ideally, once you get past your first 10+ years of practice spending, you may begin to lower your overhead to the 50-60% range, that said – it all depends on your situation and whether your focused on never-ending growth, or if you want to stabilize spending to maximize your salary.

If you see overhead at or below 50%, it is likely that the owner is under-investing and/or approaching retirement and simply trying to limit their investment due to a shorter time-horizon than you have.

You will find that most of the time, financials are explainable, but the point of looking at financials is not to walk away with a 'yes/no' opinion on a practice. What financials do is provide you a way of flagging things that require a deeper understanding from the seller. If you come away from this analysis with no questions – you're doing something wrong.

Production Analysis

As part of my analysis workbook, you will input the 10 highest production codes of the office. Spend some time understanding each of these codes as they will help you understand what type of dentistry is being done at the prospective practice.

You should see that the majority of the production is contained within the top 10 codes (60-80%) if it is less, you may be looking at a practice which is a 'jack-of-all-trades'.

Hygiene Production:

Hygiene-wise, you should expect to see 25-35% of the total production, within the Hygiene department. This is an important metric as Hygiene provides what's called 'cross-sell' – the more hygiene patients you're seeing, the higher likelihood that you are eventually going to need to complete restorative on each.

If you navigate to the FirstTimeDentist.com you'll also find a capacity utilization calculator for the Hygiene department. This portion of the workbook will help you understand how efficiently the Hygiene department is being run and/or how much 'room' you have to grow your hygiene patients without adding more clinical hours per week.

Fee Schedules:

Fees are an important part of due diligence, and one that my wife and I never really considered. While I would not recommend any immediate changes to the practice after buying (especially hiking the fees) – it is good to know how much you are over/under priced on each code.

While Fee-For-Service practices (i.e. – cash payments for all procedures up-front with no insurance / PPO reimbursements) are certainly desirable – I'm going to assume that the practice you're pursuing has some level of PPO involvement. Completing a full analysis of your PPO situation is not the intent of this document or my mission. My goal is to provide you with a basic understanding of your potential practice and some directional guidance in areas to improve. That said, services do exist to assist you with negotiating fees with PPOs (search 'Dental PPO Negotiations').

Using the evaluation workbook, you can quickly compare how the prospective practice is priced vs. the three largest PPOs. I have also built-in the ability to add market-level pricing into the workbook as well. To do so, please visit Fair Health's Fee Estimator. I purchased a fee survey for a single zip code for about $300 in 2017. While this is not absolutely necessary, it is a nice way of sizing up the overall pricing situation. For my interpretations below, I'm going to assume that you have in fact purchased this data.

Fee Evaluation

There are many factors to take into account when looking at pricing – you and your clinical abilities, punctuality, overall effectiveness, aesthetic results, patient demographics, etc. Thus, having a handle on where you are priced, relative to the market, is an important exercise.

When reviewing fees, there are three primary factors to consider – the amount ($/%) of your total production each code represents, the market price for that code, your price for that code, and the reimbursement rate of your PPOs.

Assuming that you offer a solid product (clinically) in an area of average competition, you should be charging the market rate for each code. However, even if you are charging the market rate, if your fees exceed the PPO fee schedules, you're likely to see a higher percent of write-offs in your practice (not necessarily a bad thing when managed appropriately).

Conversely, if you are priced at the market, but below the insurance fee schedule (likely to be the exception to the rule) you are not charging enough, as the PPO are willing to refund more. Depending on the production that each insurer represents – you should never be priced below the lowest PPO fee schedule as you're giving up revenue.

While there's always room for pricing optimization in the future, right now you are just trying to get a sense as to how much or little room there is to grow simply due to raising the fees. Also, you may find the Dr. has recently raised prices – are they too high? Was he trying to boost last minute production to achieve a higher price (less likely as you are looking at several years of tax returns, but who knows what he heard after that third vodka tonic at the lunch-and-learn last Friday!).

Whether your fees are too high or too low can help you explain quite a bit about the financial position in which the practice operates. Further, it may tell you more about the type of patients they attract and it serves as another sanity check. For example, if you just left an associateship where you were doing crowns at $750 a pop and this new person is charging $500 or $2,000 – you should probably raise an eyebrow to that and think 'I need to learn more.'

Reputation Research

Before you check the box on the location and financials and start spending money with your advisors, I would recommend doing some online research, if you haven't already, into the reputuation of the practice.

The purpose here is to do a small amount of leg-work to get a pulse on the profile of the owner and your prospective practice. What you are looking for is really anything that would make you do a double-take on the feasibility of purchasing the practice.

General Online Search:

What better place to start your reputation than Google[xxiv]? Simply start by typing in the Doctor's full Name. Then try their business name. What comes up? If you can't find either, just keep narrowing down your search (State, City, etc.) until you find something. If you do not find anything at all on the web about your dentist, that tells you something in-and-of-itself (no online marketing!). However, if the first thing that pops up is a mug-shot of the seller after getting a DUI a month ago, you had better believe this is going to impact the price of the practice.

Ok, so maybe the DUI example was a bit extreme and pessimistic. Let's say instead that the first thing that pops up is the doctor accepting an award for cosmetic dentistry in Switzerland. However, as part of your vision, you stated that you want to help underserved patients. Are you aligned with the business model of the practice?

As I keep saying, everything comes down to that vision of yours. Make it, use it, stick to it.

Online Reviews:

Next are good old fashioned online reviews, where anyone, from anywhere can air any dirty laundry. If you are unable to find any reviews by simply typing in the doctor's name, I would visit a few of the sites listed below and try to locate any information you can on the doctor.

Again, you're trying to establish the public image of this practice in the community. Look for reviews which speak to the level of care the doctor and staff are providing, whether the doctor's work / motives are being questioned, negative comments on the staff, etc.

> Yelp.com
> HealthGrades.com
> Vitals.com
> RateMDs.com
> Rateabiz.com

Next, we want to employ social media to find out the dirt, not just on the doctor, but on the staff. Assuming that you have the first and last names of all staff members (from Staff Survey) – you now need to perform a very technical search that most are familiar with, it is called "creeping".

Find out as much information as you can about each employee as well as the doctor. Look at their Facebook accounts, pictures they take, quotes they post ('I hate patients', 'work sucked again', #dontchoosedentistry, etc.). Again, you need to use every bit of information (especially when it is free) to help you make the biggest financial decision of your life. If you look at each of the employee's Facebooks and they are repeatedly posting negative comments about work, and the doctor tells you that the staff loves their jobs – you may want to dig a bit deeper and see if the doctor is naive to this sentiment, or if they are trying to hide something.

Do not limit your search to just Facebook, however. Look at Instagram, LinkedIn, Twitter, etc. If you can't view someone's profile because you do not have one yourself – then sign up! The internet and social media offer us an uncanny look under the hood into the culture and status of anyone, anywhere – use this to your advantage.

No detail is too small, no amount of online searching is too brash. Remember, they chose to post their profiles to the world, you're just reading their fine work. Also, do not forget that if you were to apply to a more conventional job or say even try to get a job in corporate dentistry – I would bet a month's salary that their HR department is absolutely logging into Facebook and looking at you, along with every other major corporation in America.

Note - I would be cautious on actually 'following' the practices and especially the staff that work there – as this could border a violation of your NDA if you're not discreet. Further, sites like LinkedIn allow users to view the other users who viewed their profile, so exercise caution depending on your stage in the process.

Legal Aspect:
Visit the county's court website, for the area in which your prospective practice is located. From here, you should be able to complete a search on the business. Make sure that you run several searches with the doctor's last name, business name, or any other possible aliases that may be in play.

Questions to answer include - Is the practice currently involved in a lawsuit? Have there been past complaints against the doctor? If anything does exist – has it been resolved? If you do find something but still want to pursue the practice, you should send the link to the broker and ask for an explanation (i.e. – the doctor's side of the story).

Beyond this, you can also check with the state dental board's website for the state in which the practice is located. I would do a search for any complaints or disciplinary actions taken against the doctor.

Recap

At this point you have completed an initial review on your prospective dental practice. After getting a pulse on your prospective practice, you need to decide whether to pursue this practice further. If after this chapter, you believe the practice fits your vision for your future practice, then it is time to get serious and start spending some money.

Part of the reason I have created these tools for you to use is that it allows you to survey each practice at a very high-level, before involving your accountant and lawyer. Do not misconstrue me as saying accountants and lawyers are not important to the overall process. I do believe, however, that given the right tools and background information, you are smart enough to complete a preliminary evaluation on practice leads. Hopefully you can then weed-out any less desirable practices, before spending too much time on them with your advisors.

Thus, the next logical step is to get your team involved. I would start this by sending over any and all information that your representatives. Do not hide anything from your team in this process, even what may seem like minute details of the practice could lead to your advisors being tipped off of red flags or other considerations.

After your team (primarily accountant / lawyer) receive the data, ask them for a firm time-line for them to perform their analysis and give you a preliminary view of the practice (one-to-two weeks). The accountant should be reviewing the P&L and tax returns, making adjustments and providing an overall view of their financial health. I would also request that the accountant complete a full proforma (financial projection) – assuming that you are buying the practice. Assuming that you are working with a knowledgeable accountant, ask them to perform a valuation on the dental practice as well.

Your lawyer will probably have a less tangible product; however, they should be able to at least get a general sense of the practice and its operations as well as identify any early red flags they may see. They may also recommend that you start an LLC at this point, if you have not already.

In the next chapter, we will go into a deeper level of due diligence. Here we will begin to evaluate how the practice is working from an operational perspective, survey the clinical approach and treatments, as well completing a full financial analysis.

CHAPTER 5: DUE DILIGENCE

"Money is something we trade our life's energy for."
– Henry David Thoreau

Before we jump into the details, I want to share a quick story with you. In 2016, my wife engaged a dental practice consultant. This consultant prided themselves on the sheer volume of material in which you would receive during the process. After attending an out-of-state kick-off event, we came home to a box that was so oversized, I do not think I could have wrapped my arms fully around it (and I'm 6' 5"). This box contained hundreds, no strike that, thousands of pages of manuals, instructions, checklist, procedures, forms, etc.

Now at the end of the day, this consultant definitely 'knew their stuff' and had ample experience in managing all aspects of dentistry from a business and clinical perspective. However, the thing that this consultant overlooked is that you, the dentist, the future owner, does not have the time nor the desire to read through 1,000's of pages. In fact, that is the sole purpose in which we hired the consultant, was to simplify the process.

Needless to say, this engagement ended shortly after the delivery of what could be described as the Dental Library of Congress.

My point in telling you this story is to underscore why I believe my approach will provide you value. Throughout this book, I strive to take the complex and make it simple and turn the esoteric into action. Distilling this much information down into an organized and easy to understand chapters, tools, and checklists can be a challenge. For instance, when it comes to the formal due diligence and legal process of buying a practice, there is only so much I can do to streamline it for you. It will, unfortunately, require a heavy investment of time on seemingly menial tasks, such as reviewing legal documents (yes, you too must read them), as well as a host of other tasks.

So, without further ado, let's tighten up our laces and dig in...

Financials and Valuation Overview

'Didn't we just look at financials? Why are we looking at them again?'

You probably asked yourself this question as you read the heading for this portion of the Chapter. Perhaps you even thought to yourself: 'It must be because he was a banker that he feels the need to talk about financials again.'

While I'm not going to deny that I do have a soft-spot for financial analysis, however I'm also not intending to unreasonably burden (or bore) you with inconsequential analysis.

At the end of the previous section, I recommended that you provide any and all information (primarily the Taxes and P&L) to your accountant and your lawyer. Hopefully at this point the accountant has reviewed the information and you have a time booked in your calendar to review the results. Below are some key questions that should be brought up in your discussion.

Remember, you are trying to cover three key topics with your accountant:
1. Financial Health / Performance of the Practice
2. Forward Looking Projection under your Ownership (Proforma)
3. Practice Valuation (i.e. – how much it is worth)

If your accountant does not provide these items, push them to, or get referrals from them and go find someone who will provide you the information you need (practice broker, business transition broker, etc.). I will also provide you with some basic (and free) calculators and other resources on my website, FirstTimeDentist.com.

Do note, however, when it comes to understanding the value of your practice, these tools should not replace the advice of a licensed and experienced professional, they are only meant to be supplemental and help you in the decisioning process. They are meant to help you continuously understand the desire you have to buy the practice and whether it is worthwhile or not, to continue moving forward.

Questions to Ask Your Accountant
1. Are the production/collection numbers in-line with what you would expect from a dental practice of this size (referring to patient base)?
2. Is the profitability in-line (referring to overhead)? If not, what are the major outliers?
3. At the end of the day, how much is going back into the Doctors pocket (salary, distributions, vehicles, meals, rent etc.)?
4. Do you think you can live off of this amount?
5. Do you see any red flags in the tax return filings?
6. How much is the business worth (range)?
7. Has the business been under/over-investing itself?
8. How much cash (working capital) do they recommend requesting when you start the lending process?
9. Given the valuation, what should you (the future owner) expect to make from this practice (Proforma)? (This should be after removing the loan payments which you will be required to make).
10. If the owner is paying themselves rent (via a separate business entity) is the rent amount at Fair Market Value?

Practice Valuation

Valuing a practice is difficult. Further, valuation comes in many forms, as you will see, but the one common theme is that every market is unique and has its own supply/demand dynamics. For instance, a growing midwestern city with rising wages, new job formation, and a large state university cranking out dental degrees is likely to cause for some higher competition for both patients and a practice. There are pulses here as well, while acquiring a practice might be more difficult and you may have to spend more money on getting new patients in the front door – your patients are likely to have more disposable income and be more willing/open to paying for elective treatments.

In contrast, buying a practice in an area with a low dentist / population ratio, which has no nearby dental schools and has a more challenged economic situation may prove easier to find and buy a practice. Additionally, creating a steady flow of new patients is also likely to be an easier endeavor. However, cutting all ties to PPOs or getting patients to accept comprehensive diagnoses could be a larger challenge.

Whatever market you chose, there is likely to be some level of demand for your services. Just make sure that those services are aligned with your long-term vision and can support you, financially, going forward.

In general, I highly recommend finding a dental practice broker, appraiser or accountant who has specifically worked in the area of practice valuations. In the meantime, however, please refer to my calculator on FirstTimeDentist.com which should allow you to punch in a few numbers and get a set of scenarios to consider.

I present the valuations in the form of a bell-curve distribution chart, as I want to be clear – there is no single price that is 'correct'. Just like searching for a home, you may find a home you're willing to make an offer on, but only a 'low-ball' offer. In contrast, a person may find that this same home is exactly what they have been searching for and are willing to pay more than the asking price. Who was paying the 'right' price? Neither. They were both attempting to assign value to the practice, based on their perceptions of layout, color, location, and proximity to work.

In this sense, I want you to use each of the follow methods of my valuation spreadsheet to estimate a ballpark cost for the practice. As you learn more and develop a deeper opinion, this viewpoint will certainly change. Without walking you through an undergraduate level course in corporate finance, I did want to briefly explain my two approaches.

Market Valuation:

This approach basically says, how much does the practice produce in a year, and by how much do we need to 'value' those cash flows. For instance, if your potential practice makes $1mm / year in gross revenues, and you have a market valuation ratio of 60%, you would expect to pay in the ball park of $600k. Could be more or less, based on the location, the 'newness' of the equipment, etc.

Discounted Cash Flows:

This is a much more traditional and academic approach to practice valuations. Essentially it says that 'todays' dollars are worth more than money earned in the future (i.e. – I would rather have $100 today than $125 in 5 years). It then requires that you project forward your future practice's cash flows and 'discount' these cash flows back to today's dollars.

Real Estate

If you are also considering purchasing the land/building associated with the practice, you will run into a similar valuation issue. Unlike the practice valuation, however, there is typically no cash flow that you would receive from the real estate (unless you plan on becoming a landlord, which would possibly negate the need to be a dentist!). Thus, Real Estate is worth whatever the market is willing to pay for it.

I would recommend also finding a certified commercial real estate appraiser or broker to provide you with either a full appraisal (costlier but should be more accurate) OR a BOV (broker opinion of value), which should be faster and cheaper but possibly have more 'variance' built-into them.

Similar to the practice valuations, I have created a spreadsheet which will give you the ability to get a rough estimate of a fair price for your building.

Capitalization ("Cap") Rate:

Essentially, this method looks at the cost of leasing a facility and the required rate of return for a landlord. The higher the rate of return, the lower the cost of the building needed to achieve that rate (keeping the building price the same).

You can, in turn, use this rate to estimate the cost of buying the building, given the required rate of return by the market.

Cost / Square Foot:

More simplistic, but still reasonable approach, you can look at the cost / square foot of other buildings of similar size, usage, location, etc. and compare that to your building. If you are choosing to lease a building, I have also created a quick spreadsheet which will allow you to pull in 'comps' and compare it to your own prospective location.

Note – do ensure that your lawyer reads through any existing lease agreements between the current owner and landlord. Some leases could have 'kick-out' clauses which allow the landlord to 'kick-out' a tenant, should they sell their business. It could force you to renegotiate with the landlord, which puts you at a disadvantage as they will be keenly aware that you're unlikely to want to buy a practice and immediately move it.

You're probably wondering where you will get all this real estate information? I would recommend starting with LoopNet.com or looking for a local Commercial Real Estate (CRE). You will likely find a handful of both national and local CRE firms, try taking a look at their websites for a list of properties and sale prices. If you live in a smaller town, you can try contacting the largest local residential realtor as they have likely done some CRE deals themselves. Do note, LoopNet.com is attempting to be the 'Zillow' of the commercial real estate space. Some will argue that true commercial real estate is exchanged 'off market' between parties who have existing business relationships. Therefore, the only remaining properties (i.e. – 'scraps') get listed on the site. I would argue that this is not entirely true and to just keep these points in perspective.

Keep in mind, the goal of buying a practice should not be to get the best deal I the world, but to find and create your place in the world. If you walk away thinking that you got a screaming deal, it is likely that you either didn't fully account for some of the inherent risks, or you just made an enemy of the former doctor.

Engaging Your Team

At this point in the process, you should start working more closely with the remainder of your team (outside your lawyer and accountant). You will need to kick off the lending process, begin getting quotes on insurance rates, starting a business with your lawyer, and finding a bank. Please refer back to Chapter 2: Building Your Team for a list of common questions that you should be asking when considering each company.

Legal

Start by ensuring your lawyer has all the necessary documents needed to review the potential practice. Documents like leases, easements, or other ancillary agreements between the seller and other parties should be reviewed immediately. If you have not completed it, also ask that your lawyer complete a quick search for any historical or outstanding litigations against the selling doctor.

As I mentioned, if your location is leased, ensure that the lawyer spends an adequate amount of time reviewing the lease to ensure you can acquire this document without any major hiccups.

Have your lawyer touch base with your accountant to discuss the best corporate structure (from a tax perspective) for your business. While everyone is unique and could potentially have a different recommendation, the vast majority of dentists will likely land in an LLC (Limited Liability Company[xxv]). What you need to know is this – choosing a company type is very important (would not recommend doing this by yourself). It can protect you both legally and financially. Having an LLC shifts the liability (if the business is run correctly and the 'Corporate Veil' is not 'Pierced'[xxvi]) to the business vs. you personally.

In addition, you can elect to be taxed as an LLC or and LLC doing business as an S-Corp[xxvii]. Without getting too deep into the details, an S-Corp can be beneficial in allowing you to take home additional profits in the form of distributions (cash paid to you directly out of business without standard payroll deductions). This can allow you to save on Social Security and Medicare taxes. This is far from a panacea, however, there are multiple things I'm glossing over (minimum salary must be met first, federal taxes paid at year-end on distributions, etc.) for which you should discuss further with your accountant.

Get Your Lenders Involved

If at this point you haven't already started the lending process with your bank, I would contact them to get this process started. Essentially, they will ask that you fill out a detailed application with a host of data requests, to get the process started.

Most of it will be personal information to allow them to pull your credit history and begin to form their opinion on your credit worthiness.

After which, you will need to send them the same detailed information that you have sent to your accountant and your lawyer (P&L, Production Reports, Tax Returns, etc.). You still have some time as you will need to still negotiate the price and sign a Letter of Intent, but I to introduce the concept now.

Ensure that you're working with 2-3 lenders, in case one decides to back out of the deal, or does not approve you, you will save yourself some heartache by having another lender 'teed-up'. In our experience, the broker was very confident that a regional bank would easily approve the loan, they didn't, due to my wife's lack of experience in owning a business. This stemmed from the bank having lost money recently on a practice which was purchased and subsequently failed. Thankfully, I had not one, but two additional lenders in which we could review their offers.

Insurance Agent

Through either online searches or referrals, find a local insurance agent who offers both P&C (Property and Casualty) and Dental Malpractice Insurance, at a minimum. You will likely need life, disability, and overhead insurance in the future – but save that for Year 1 of owning your practice.

Note – sometimes life insurance is required to finalize the closure with your lender, ask your lender EARLY if this is required as Life Insurance underwriting can take weeks or months and require significant paperwork, medical evaluations (in person), as well as phone calls/interviews.

The main thing to ask for here is a quote, similar to auto or home insurance, on what your premiums will be (payments) and what type / amount of insurance you will receive in return. On the P&C side, the agent will likely be interested in the amount of fixed assets the business owns, whether the building is owned/leased, how large the building is, and different practice and building characteristics.

In terms of malpractice insurance, there are two main terms to become acquainted with: Claims-Made and Occurrence. I will refer you to PSIC's[xxviii] website (not necessarily an endorsement, just a good description), or your agent for additional details. High-level, the Claims-Made covers you only during a covered period (unless 'Tail' Coverage is purchased).

Conversely, Occurrence Malpractice Insurance 'kicks-in' and covers you for any situations which occur currently or during the past, without the purchase of 'Tail' coverage. I would encourage you to discuss this topic thoroughly with your agent, and make sure that if you do decide to pursue the former 'Claims-Made' that you are aware of the risks and your own personal work history.

In terms of coverage limits, the limit is usually quoted in two amounts: $1mm/$2mm and $2mm/$4mm. What the first number stands for is the amount you will be covered for any once single incident, while the second number is your maximum for all incidents.

Banking

You can argue to open a bank account early, for convenience and one less thing to do later, or you could argue to let it be a bargaining chip with the lender (i.e. – 'if I bring my full banking relationship to you, can I get a discount on my loan?'). Given that not all dental lenders will have a physical branch near you (or even in your state, in my case) – you may want to consider separating the lending from the banking aspect. Keep in mind, it is not too difficult to shut down a bank account if you do decide to move your primary banking relationship to your lender.

As mentioned, I would recommend opening both a checking and a savings account and putting a few thousand dollars in each to start. Yes, this does come out of your personal pocket and should be something you make aware to the accountant. It makes it much easier, in my opinion, when you can start moving all your expenses on behalf of the business into the business, vs. spending out of your personal pocket and then trying to keep track of them for later use.

Site Visit

Prior to making an offer, I would recommend setting up time with the broker / doctor to complete a site visit. This may very well be the first time you meet either of these individuals in person, so make the most of the trip. I would setup an entire day (you do not want to be rushed) to complete the on-site due diligence.

There are three important reasons for seeing the practice in-person:
1. Evaluation of Facilities
2. Evaluation of Equipment / Post Closing Equipment Needs
3. Chart Review

Below is a proposed schedule for your site visit at the office. You're likely to need one full day, so I would plan-out the day and provide it in writing to the broker/doctor in advance. The point of this visit is to see things from the eyes of the doctor, in terms of both equipment and patient records. Additionally, it offers the chance to interview the doctor and get direct answers to any questions that bubble-up throughout the day.

Proposed Schedule for Day:

Arrive: 9:00 am

Get there early, but not too early. You want to see how serious the seller is, if they are not willing to be there at 9am on their day off, it could make you question the seriousness of the seller and their desire to go through with the transition. Also, make note of whether the Doctor (and broker if they are coming) show up on time. If not, record how many minutes they were late.

Office Tour: 9:00 – 9:30am

After exchanging pleasantries, ask the Doctor to give you a tour of the office. This will help acclimate you to the office as well as break the ice. This, of course, may not be necessary if you already completed the mystery shop exercise in Chapter 4).

Checklists: 9:30 – 11:30am

After the tour, politely let the doctor know that you have a long set of checklists that you want to run through which involve walking through the office/operatories, inspecting equipment, and thoroughly reviewing charts. How does the Doctor respond? Are they hesitant? You should have 100% full access to anything and everything you need during due diligence, do not take 'no' for an answer. After this, begin your checklists for the Evaluation of Facilities and Equipment Inventory.

Chart Evaluation: 11:30am – 12:30pm

Using the Chart Evaluation workbook, complete random chart reviews on roughly 10% of the active patients (see below for what to look for).

Lunch with Doctor: 12:30 – 2:00pm

Make plans, in advance, for lunch with the Doctor. This can be a very informal way of getting to know them, they are personality, how they run the practice, etc. Also, it affords you the immediate opportunity to ask questions on anything that stuck out to you in the initial checklist process. Did you see something that didn't make sense to you in your initial chart review? Ask! Again, they should be an 'open-book' if they truly want to sell. Depending on the Doctor, they may try to buy you lunch, certainly take it if offered, but if they at all hesitate when the server comes to you, do ask for separate checks (and note that fact that the Doctor wants you to spend $500k of money you do not have and they didn't want to buy you a $12 hamburger).

Chart Evaluation Continued: 2:00 – 3:30 (or 4:00) pm

Continue chart reviews until finishing with ~10% of patients. Once you've complete this you may have the opportunity to ask just a few more questions to the doctor before departing. I would keep them light as you have taken quite a bit of their time at this point. However, since you have things fresh in your mind and you have the doctor in front of you, take advantage of the opportunity.

Later that Evening

Once you get home, but before you turn on TV and relax, spend just a few minutes documenting your day. Type up a list of questions for your lawyer/accountant (before you forget them). You might even consider making a document which serves as a running list of questions (and answers) that you can take with you throughout the process. Do also take the time to send a personalized letter (or e-mail) to the seller, as they did welcome you into their practice for a day.

Evaluation of Facilities

Similar to the approach we took when evaluating the location and exterior of the facilities, you also need to take a similar approach on the interior. Below is a list of items to look at while in the office. Make sure you look at all the details you can, take notes, take pictures, even take a video as you may need it later.

Basic Information:

Number of Computers: _____
Computer in Every Operatory? _____
Software System / Version: _____
Paper Filing System (Yes/No): _____

Appearance: _____ (report card scale: A-F)

What to look for: As you walk up to the building what do you notice? Is it the landscaping (if any) clean and taken care of? When you walk through the front door, what is your first impression? Is there plenty of natural light? Sticky notes everywhere? Professional looking? Needing repairs?

Furniture and Fixtures:_____ (report card scale: A-F)

What to look for: What is the condition of the overall office, in terms of its furniture and fixtures (lighting, cabinetry, art, other decorations).? What is the condition of the carpeting/flooring? Is there plenty of lighting throughout? Would any of it need replaced post-close? It would be good to jot down anything you would replace.

Organization: _____ (report card scale: A-F)

What to look for: One of the biggest assets your buying is Goodwill – which is an intangible asset which is meant to measure the innate ability of patients to keep coming back and your team to keep providing services to them. My point is that if the office is messy, unorganized, and cluttered, this should affect the purchase price. Look at the front desk, is it clean and organized, or does it have piles of papers and notes? Go into the lab, sterilization and a few of the operatories and open the cabinets – is everything labeled? Does every inventory item have a place? Go into the backroom, Dr.s' office, etc. and look for signs of clutter, dirt, or anything else that demonstrates a lack of systems.

Floorplan: _____ (report card scale: A-F)

What to look for: How do you feel about the layout of the practice? Is it spacious or cramp? Do operatories face the exterior of the building (allowing the Dr. and staff to move freely in the hallway without having to say 'hi' to every patient)? Are there one or two entrances into each operatory (two allows the dentist to enter one and assistant to enter the other)? Ergonomics of the lab? How is the Drs.' office setup vs. what you would expect? Is the sterilization room centrally located? Is there an employee break-room?

Compliance: _____ (report card scale: A-F)

What to look for: Does the office appear to be following OSHA standards? Is the sterilization up to code? Do you see any violations of HIPPA? Does the office appear to meet ADA (Americans with Disabilities Act)? On-site clothes laundering? Are there wheelchair ramps, bathrooms with grab bars, room underneath sink, wide doorways, etc.?

Equipment Checklist

As mentioned above in the proposed schedule, I recommend taking a good hour or so to go through each operatory to review the equipment. You're, first, looking to an assessment of the general condition of the existing equipment. Beyond that, you should use the detailed checklist (FirstTimeDentist.com) to help you track the items that you will need to purchase, post close, as well as any items which may need replaced in the near future. Having a documented list of existing/needed equipment helps you in two ways. First, it can play a role into the valuation of the practice – if the practice feels to be too pricey, but it is filled with brand new equipment you might be able to stomach the cost. Secondly, if you do move into the 'execution' phase, you will want to place your equipment orders in advance of the close date.

It may seem odd, my recommendation to buying equipment right out of the gate, however sometimes you will have a skill or interest in performing certain procedures or techniques the old doctor did not complete. For my wife, she was used to doing extractions on a regular basis, due to her year in residency. The owner of the practice she bought did not have the oral surgery handpieces and equipment necessary to complete these procedures. Alternatively, make sure you are comfortable with the brand and type of instruments and equipment used in the office. If you simply have experience on a different set of equipment, you may want to consider replacing it immediately. Remember, your product is your clinical work – you want to avoid delivering substandard products due to unfamiliarity with the tools of the trade.

Chart Evaluation

Reviewing charts may seem like an arduous task, and it is. My hope is, however, that with a little background information and, you guessed it, another tool on FirstTimeDentist.com that I can make this process as efficient as possible for you.

Remember, these charts will be your gateway into understating patient's clinical history. It is important that you understand the notes, clinical approach, and outcome for past procedures.

In general, the point of reviewing charts is to begin to get a clinical understanding of the patients and the treatments the current doctor is prescribing. The goal is to review 10% of the active patient's base. Some individuals recommend physically counting a portion of the charts (if paper ones even exist in this practice) and then doing some quick math to estimate the number of active patients. Personally, I'll trust their dental software's estimate on the number of patients seen in the last 12-18 months.

But what are you actually looking for when you review charts? You should be treating each chart as 'desk treatment plan'. In that, you do not have the benefit of the patient sitting in front of you, you only have the X-Rays, patient appointment history, and doctor notes at your disposal. You want to review each restorative case and ask yourself whether the doctor was being too aggressive? Too conservative? Is there remaining work to be done or have all the cavities and crowns that need done, have been done?

If you find yourself constantly challenging the doctor's diagnoses, you should take note as this could be a problem down the road. If the doctor is unusually aggressive in their treatments and you are more conservative – patients may think you do not know what you're doing or that you do not care as much. Conversely, if the previous doctor was very conservative and rarely prescribed treatments of a certain type – you may get some resistance from patients when your treatment plan as they may think the new doctor is trying to 'pay off their loans'.

I saw a great quote on LinkedIn the other day. The gist was... "If you want to make people happy, be an Ice Cream Man. If you want to change the world, become a leader". Point is, at the end of the day, you will never make everyone happy and that's certainly not what I'm prescribing here. What you do need to walk away with is a clear grasp on what you're getting yourself into. Again, everything plays into the price that you're willing to pay.

Additionally, you're also trying to get a general sense of how much dentistry is 'left'? In that, if you have 1,000 patients and the majority of the patients are in bite splints, have several crowns, implants, or dentures – is there anything left for you?

Obviously, teeth will break over-time, crowns will come off, and new cavities will form and hopefully there is a steady stream of new patients. However, you can't tell the bank to just wait for their payment as you saw a patient at the grocery store walking out with 3 cases of Mountain Dew. If you do find serious limitations in the amount of work in the existing patient base, you may need to consider additional marketing approaches to bring in more new patients to begin treatment planning.

I would recommend that you visit FirstTimeDentist.com and search for the Chart Evaluation tool. The tool is designed to create an efficient means by which to survey the charts, collect information, and ultimately understand the clinical inner-workings of this office.

Business Operations Evaluation

I'll say it again, because it is just this important, the majority of what you're buying is a fictitious, esoteric asset called 'goodwill'. It represents the proclivity of patients to continue their past behaviors of going to your office, as well as the operations and systems in place to service those patients.

Earlier, I made reference to one of my favorite books of all-time "E-Myth Revisited" by Michael Gerber. His book is focused solely on you, the entrepreneur, and helping you attain as successful of a life as you want, with as limited pain points as possible. In order to do so, he preaches the never-ending process of creating and refining 'systems'. Note – I would not recommend the Dental Version of the E-Myth due to it being written by two dentists from the UK. The story is much more impactful in the E-Myth Revisited shown above.

But, what is a Business 'System'?

A system is any set of tools you use to manage your business, so as to provide as seamless, efficient, and consistent product or service to your customers. Again, not referring to IT systems here. We're talking about checklists, employee procedures (sterilization, room setup) or patient interactions.

I think it is best to demonstrate this concept with a real-time example. The next time you go to your favorite local restaurant, I want you to take some time and watch closely the staff and how they work. For example, you walk into the restaurant and you are typically greeted by a smiling host or hostess. They ask you the number of people in your party and then they go find and prepare your table. Upon returning, the host(ess) then walks you to your table, seats you and introduces your server's name.

At some point the server comes over with some waters for the table, takes a drink order, then returns with the drinks and takes your dinner order. Lastly, your food is delivered by a runner (not the server) once complete. Your server usually checks-in with the table a few more times to make sure nothing else is needed, water glasses are full, and to take the check.

Now let's compare this to a restaurant without any systems. You walk into the restaurant and wait 5-10 minutes with multiple staff members walking past you. Finally, just as you are about to flag someone down, a server stops and asks 'have you been helped yet'? You tell them it is a party of two and they shrug and say 'just a minute'. Five minutes later a different server comes over and walks you to your table. They take your drink order and leave.

Next, your drinks are delivered by the host(ess), however one of the drinks is wrong. You suggest that you ordered a Martini, not an Old Fashioned; dumbfounded the host(ess) says "Okay…let me go talk to the bartender." Then, you wait… in uncomfortable silence as your spouse sips their drink and you do not have one. Now you've waited 5-10 minutes to get in, received the wrong drink, didn't receive the correct drink, and you're starving.

I'm sure you have had an experience or two like this at a restaurant or other business establishment. What went wrong? They may have had the correct staff in the right positions – but they were not assigned specific roles and/or they didn't follow those roles.

If your potential practice does not have clear, concise, and updated job descriptions, procedures, etc. you will be in eternal job confusion purgatory. When employees do not know whose job it is, things get forgotten, assumed, or worse ignored. Most likely, if you're purchasing a practice from an older dentist who has been working in the same building for 25 or 30 years – they are unlikely to have a set of updated and modern operations which govern your day-to-day productivity. While this certainly not a deal breaker – it is, again, something to consider when trying to assign a value to the practice.

So how do we know if the existing Doctor has a solid set of systems? You will probably have to do some digging, unless of course they have shared a detailed list of procedures, job descriptions, etc.

Below is a list of questions that you need to answer. Remember, you are buying a business and that business should run whether you're at the helm, the old dentist, or a dentist from the other end of the country. Make sure you get answers to all of these questions throughout the due diligence process:

General:
1. Who is in charge of opening/closing the office each day?
2. Who is in charge of ordering dental supplies? Office supplies?
3. Is there a digital back-up process?
4. Is there someone 'on point' for handling OSHA/HIPPA Compliance?
5. Does the dentist have a spouse or family member working in the practice? If so, what is their role (specific details here)?
6. Is everything labeled throughout the practice (sundries, dental equipment, front desk, office supplies, etc.)?

Financial:
1. Who does the day-to-day bookkeeping for the practice (i.e. – 'QuickBooks')?
2. Who is in charge of processing/following-up on insurance reimbursements?
3. Is there a written policy for financial arrangements?
4. Does the front desk balance and close-out the account each day?
5. Who pays invoices, credit card bills, utilities, etc.?
6. Who takes cash/check deposits to the bank?

Quick Tip – *if you ask employees to do this on behalf of the company, the company can be liable if the employee is in an accident on the way to the bank – check with your lawyer for more information.*

Insurance:
1. Who submits? How (electronic, hopefully...)?
2. Who follow-ups with issues?
3. Who is in charge of collections?
4. Is there a written process for collections?
5. Do they use an attorney or collection agency for past due accounts?

Marketing:
1. Where does the current dentist advertise?
2. Does the dentist do any Direct Mail marketing?
3. Does the dentist pay for any SEO (search engine optimization) or other digital advertising?
4. What does the dentist's social media presence look like? Do they advertise here?
5. Does the dentist use an appointment reminder service?

Facility Maintenance:
1. Who cuts grass / takes care of landscaping (where applicable)?
2. Who is in charge of plowing snow (where applicable)?
3. Who is in charge of cleaning floors, bathrooms, windows, etc.?
4. Who is responsible for dental equipment cleaning (filters, traps, etc.)?
5. Who is in charge of general building maintenance?
6. Who is in charge of general dental equipment maintenance?

Clinical:
1. Post-Op Instructions written and ready to be handed out?
2. Written consent forms ready to be signed?
3. Procedure quotation system (how are quotes delivered to patients?
4. Note taking - Doctor or Staff (Who?)? How often (daily, weekly?)
5. Extent of Content (are notes extremely detailed or on the lighter side)?
6. Established tray setups / needed instruments for each procedure for both restorative and hygiene appointments?
7. What are the sterilization procedures? OSHA compliant?

Other Systems:
1. Are their written procedures for the front desk, assistants, hygiene, etc.?
2. Do employees have written copies of their job descriptions?

3. Does the front desk 'screen' patients before putting them on the schedule?
4. Does the front desk track referrals?
5. Are employees cross-trained at all (the more, the better)?
6. Does the front desk have any scripting for new patients, appointments being cancelled, etc.?
7. Who maintains HIPAA / OSHA compliance manuals? MSDS's? How often?
8. Are there new hire / termination / retirement procedures?

Most offices have 'people' instead of 'processes'. What I mean by that is, when a question arises about how to do some task, we say 'go ask Sally at the front desk'. Instead of, 'what does the systems manual say'. Our goal is to take the people out of this scenario, as people come and go. People get sick, have major life events, etc. The more you rely on a single person vs. a process, the more you become an indentured servant to that person performing the task(s) assigned as well as showing up each day to work.

The point of having systems in place is to also provide absolute clarity on who owns what tasks, how exactly to do the tasks, and how often the tasks need completed. This section should help you size up the effort needed to get these systems in place in your potential practice. Additionally, have as much documentation as possible can help, should any of your staff decide to leave rather quickly upon your acquisition of the practice.

I would fully expect that the majority of the practices you look at will likely be run using the 'people' model instead of the 'process'. Sure, there may be a handful of items that are documented in a miscellaneous or disorderly manner. What we will want to strive for, however, is an office where everyone has the inherent knowledge or ability to complete anyone else's tasks (within the extent of the law obviously).

For my wife, she purchased a practice which, not surprisingly, had little systems in place. The practice relied heavily on the daily involvement of both the doctor and the doctor's spouse. While the practice was efficiently run, had strong profit margins, and a regimented approach to the daily grind – it was not a sustainable process.

We believe that the doctor put too much stress on himself by taking control of any and all details. Eventually, we think the level of stress the doctor was under eventually may have caused him to retire 3-5 years earlier than he may have otherwise. While this may come across as a benefit, we need to think larger picture – we want you to enjoy your job so much that you work as long as you chose.

Thus, do not despair when your practice has a 'name' listed against every task, just note that this is going to be something which requires significant work in the first few years.

Teaser – I'm hoping to follow this book up with a second book, focusing on how to thrive in your first year of practice. I believe systems are going to be a crucial component of this book as they were one of the biggest struggles for my wife. Many consultants exist to help you build and implement such systems in your practice. We have dealt with a handful and have strong opinions on each. My advice, ensure that you do your research, get references, and have a clear plan (presented to you) prior to signing any contracts with a consultant. Also make sure there is an 'out' in the contract, should you decide that things are not going as expected (we exercised our 'out' half-way through a rather expensive consulting arrangement).

Staff Evaluation and Salaries

While we're in the habit of combing through the details on work flow, job descriptions and roles at the practice – it only makes sense to examine each of the staff members and their respective pay.

Staff Evaluations:

The goal of this exercise is to get an inventory of the employees, their general job descriptions, and their value to the company. Visit FirstTimeDentist.com to get your copy of the evaluation worksheet. Do note, it is quite possible that the broker/seller has already completed a similar exercise. However, I wanted to make sure you at least had a template to send over and formally request the information, if not readily provided.

Most of the columns are pretty self-explanatory, up until the last two. While there are many ways of assessing a person's performance or value to a company, I found this method to be the most interesting. Some consultants refer to this as a '9 box', basically a 3 x 3 matrix with the employee's potential on the X-axis and Performance on the Y-axis.

The goal of this exercise is to establish not only how each employee is performing today, but what their true potential is. As you get deeper into business ownership you will learn that star players are not born, they are bred. You need to find people with the right attitude, solid technical skills, and a superb willingness to learn can be coached into one of your strongest assets. If you have a team of 'C' players, but all have the potential to be 'A', you should be thrilled as you do not have to wait for them to leave (or fire them) in order to upgrade their skill sets.

In terms of the 'Low-Low's – I hope that no dental practice has any of these individuals working for you, but if they do – you will need to push hard on them to improve, otherwise you may need to consider parting ways with them (if they truly are 'Low-Low'), and quickly. Bad employees with negative attitudes are like a cancer, unchecked, they will spread amongst your entire team. People then start lowering their standards of work to this individual, instead of raising their standards to the highest performer in the office.

Staff Salary Survey:

I have created a quick tool which allows you to compare data from Salary.com or Indeed.com (free salary information for your prospective area) to what the employees are currently being paid. In general, you probably want to be closer to the median than you are to either the top or bottom end, unless your practice vision is situated on either of these tails.

Do not forget that the hourly rate is only part of the compensation. As you see above you can also compensate employees through paid time-off, holidays, uniform allowance, year-end bonuses, health insurance, dental procedure discounts, etc. Make sure that you take these points into account as you compare their salaries to the averages.

Spouses & Family Members:

In the course of reviewing employee roster, you may discover that there is a spouse, child or other relative of the doctor's working in the practice. Even if they are not physically 'in' the practice on a daily basis, it is common that the dentist's spouse is involved in some way in the practice (I do the accounting, legal, and other administrative tasks for my wife).

There are two issues with this scenario. First, you need to ensure that there are no expectations that the spouse expects to retain employment post-closing. Barring any extreme situations, I would generally urge you to cut the cord on any such circumstances quickly.

The issue is that, similar to working with the closing dentist during a 'phase-out' period – you're likely to experience some level of conflict. You likely perceive there to be a litany of changes that need to be made, and the existing doctor (or spouse) may disagree with these changes, as they have been 'doing it this way for years.'

The second, and more likely, scenario is that the spouse of the doctor is paying the bills, submitting insurance, doing payroll, or completing other administrative tasks. The concern here is that these tasks can be underrepresented in your analysis of the income statement and hours that the employees work.

Often, spouses are either not being paid or, if they are compensated, not being paid for the hours in which they contribute. Thus, if you are taking over a practice where the doctors spouse is spending 10 hours a week doing administrative tasks – you now have a decision to make. Do you (or your spouse) take over these tasks, requiring you find additional time in your busy schedules? Or, do you outsource these tasks to accountants, bookkeepers, or your staff? Either options are likely to add costs and/or unforeseen headaches.

I would urge you to get a detailed list of tasks (and hours spent / frequency of tasks) which are completed by the dentist's family member. You want this list to be as specific as possible so that you can properly account for this time and money in your forecasted P&L.

Employee Manual:

If your prospective practice has an employee manual, do try to get your hands on a copy of it. The employee manual may set the stage for the type of management style the doctor exhibits (a 300-page detailed document may show signs of a micromanager). The manual will also give you a documented understanding that exists between both the employees and the business. It will help you develop an awareness on the employee benefits, vacation policy, bonus policy, etc.

Ideally, as a business owner someday, you will have an employee manual in place for two reasons. First, it provides a written contract, if you will, between the business and employees – detailing what they are entitled to if they complete their roles effectively. Secondly, this document provides some legal protection / risk mitigation for the owner. For instance, if you feel the need to terminate an employee, when you can point back to the manual and show that you agreed to these terms and the violation is cause for dismal.

Note: Writing an employee manual by yourself is both an intimidating and legally dicey endeavor. It is extremely easy to make a statement such as 'overtime will not be paid for continuing education trips'. Please know that the laws governing employee / business relationships are quite specific. Documenting that your practice is choosing not to follow federal, state, or local laws is essentially and up-front admission of guilt. There are plenty of legally-backed employee manual / HR services available. Do some research and make sure that they allow for customization (you do not want a stock template like we were suckered into at one point).

Bringing it All Together

Hopefully by the end of this Chapter, you will have developed a deep understanding of the inner-workings of your prospective dental practice. You should have a firm grasp on the overall strength of the financials, systems, and the employees.

How do you boil all this down into a single 'go' / 'no-go' decision on the practice however? There are two approaches to consider to help you 'frame-up' what the desirability of the practice.

SWOT Analysis

You can get a piece of paper, or even a napkin for that matter and draw four large boxes. Below is a simple example of a SWOT analysis that you can conduct in relatively short order. The point is to put all the qualitative measures on a single page, step back and take a strategic view of this practice. Does it make sense that you can overcome the weakness and turn them into opportunities, while guarding against your strengths becoming threats?

Practice Strengths	Practice Weaknesses
-Large Patient Base	-Lack of Business Systems
-Strong Demographics	-Poor Location
-Experienced Employees	-Poor Floorplan
Practice Opportunities	Practice Threats
-Ordering Efficiencies	-New Practice Nearby
-Additional Marketing	-Road Construction

Scorecard Analysis:

At the end of the day, the decision to fully pursue a practice is going to be based on a collection of mostly qualitative factors. There is no special equation, formula or statistical model that can be applied. Thus, my approach would be to line-up all the factors that matter most to you and simply grade each one. This can be a check-mark, an "X", numbers, letters – doesn't really matter. The point is, you want to look back at all you've analyzed throughout this book and sum up each section into a single value. Doing so, will allow you to see everything on one page. If you see two check marks in the financials, but everything else has a large red "X", then you have to seriously consider whether that one category is enough to outweigh the remaining.

FIRST TIME DENTIST

Scorecard

Topic	Score *Whatever metric you would like*	Notes
Employees *Strong workers? Risk in leaving?*		
Business Systems *Organized workflow?*		
Location / Facilities *Desirable? Needs work?*		
Financials *Strong? Weak? Not Adding up?*		
Fits Lifestyle *Is this what you really want?*		
Cost *Are you comfortable with it?*		
Demographics *Type of Patients you want to serve?*		
Business Model *FFS vs. PPO vs. Medicaid*		
Other Topics		

Recap

In this chapter, we took a deep dive into due diligence. We visited the practice for some hands-on evaluations of patient files, equipment and the facility itself. You analyzed the staff, their roles, the overall operations/systems of the business and spent some additional time looking at valuations. Lastly, you took all the data you have accumulated up unto this point and used it to come up with a single recommendation ('go'/'no-go'). You should feel proud, this was a ton of work!

In Chapter 6, we will assume that you are moving forward with your prospective practice. We will begin the negotiation process, walking you through the various stages and levers in which you can use to craft the deal. Remember, the deal is about more than the price!

CHAPTER 6: NEGOTIATIONS

"What would you do if you weren't afraid?"
– 'Who Moved my Cheese' (Spencer Johnson)

You've made it to Chapter 6, and we're finally going to start negotiating! For some people, negotiating provides a sense of euphoria. They love getting into combat mode, strapping up their boots and digging in their heels. However, for the majority of people – negotiating elicits a different response.

I'm hoping that you've purchased some larger-sized item at some point in your life (house, car, motorcycle, condo, etc.). If so, the process of negotiating for a dental practice should seem familiar.

I think about negotiations in five stages:
1. "Getting-to-Know You": this is the part where you exchange pleasantries with the seller (or broker) you discuss your background, your goals, etc. This is basically the entire Due Diligence phase that we just discussed
2. Making an Offer: this will come in the form of a Letter of Intent (LOI)
3. Accepting the Offer: this is usually done with the LOI through several rounds of 'back-and-forth' between buyer and seller
4. Negotiating the Agreements: after the agreement is done, this will kick-off a whole new round of legal work on either side
5. Finalizing the Agreements / Closing: this is the final step in 'dotting the I's and crossing the T's' on the agreements and then preparing for the closing day for the practice transfer.

You have already completed the "Getting-to-Know You" stage if you have made it this far in your due diligence. Thus, for this Chapter, we will focus on #2-4 above, with some additional information on financing your practice. #5 (Finalizing the Agreements) will be covered in our last Chapter "Closing".

Making an Offer

To 'get the ball rolling' on this practice, you will likely need to make the first move in the negotiation process – making an offer. The key to this process, in my opinion, is to move fast. During my wife's transition, we had quite a few hang-ups with our advisors which, for one reason or another, which caused us to delay making an offer for several weeks. We actually received a personal call from the seller asking us if we were still interested / planning on making an offer. This was both frustrating and embarrassing the LOI should have been assembled, delivered, and responded to in the time it took us to just assemble it.

The punch-line is – if you know you want this practice, if it is fits your criteria and you haven't found any red flags yet – you have got make an offer and quick. Make sure you have mutually agreed-upon deadlines with your advisors (most items should be reviewed / returned to you within a few days, no longer than a week). This shows the broker and seller that you are serious and will at least 'get your hat in the ring' should any other buyers show up looking to purchase as well. Had my wife been dealing with a doctor who hadn't seemingly already made up his mind about who he would sell to, she easily could have lost the practice to another buyer, due to our delays.

Negotiating Levers

While the price of the practice is certainly going to be the biggest driver of your (and the seller's) agreement, there are several other components of the deal that should be considered. Below is a list of some common and less-common 'levers' you can use to negotiate. Remember, you can't pursue every one of the items I have listed below. The goal is to find (through the negotiation process) the items in which the seller is more or less sensitive. You need to think creatively in the process about how you can extract value in other parts of this transaction, outside of price.

Seller Financing:

Consider asking the seller to finance part of the practice loan (working capital?). Working with the seller in this way can benefit both you and the seller.

For you (the buyer) you again get some peace of mind that the seller has a vested interest in your success as defaulting on your loan will only cause headaches for them.

For the seller, they can extend their current ownership of the real estate into an on-going cash stream. For instance, if they chose to do a 10-year seller financing loan, the seller may be able to either supplement or replace the need to take cash out of their retirement for some period of time. This gives them piece of mind, as they enter retirement. Additionally, the seller delays the bulk influx of cash (due to a sale), which allows them to possibly reduce their capital gains in the same year that they will (hopefully) see a gain on the sale of their practice, possibly pushing them into a higher tax bracket.

This can also send a signal to the owner and reinforce the need of them to ensure the transition goes well – as they have a vested interest in you succeeding, after the sale.

While seller financing on the practice loan is usually not the norm (due to the preponderance of low cost lending from large institutions), you can also consider it on Real Estate. If the seller happens to own his or her building (and you want to buy it) I would highly recommend pursuing this option. Commercial Real Estate (CRE) loans may prove to be more difficult, in terms of acquiring financing from a bank. At a minimum, they certainly will require more up front due diligence (appraisal, survey, Phase I/II, etc.), and may require that the seller put down additional funds as a down payment.

Balloon Loans:

Balloon Loans are essentially a way of achieving lower payments (by stretching the <u>amortization</u> of your loan over a longer time period) but not commit the lender to a long-term loan. Essentially, you can take out a loan by which payments are calculated on a 15-year amortization schedule (length of loan) but have a balloon payment in Year 5 for the outstanding balance of the loan.

I hesitated mentioning these loans as they can be dangerous. However, I feel strongly about being transparent in the actions we took and the pros/cons of each choice. Further, my goal is to simply present everything that should be in your toolkit, not everything works for everyone. Thus, if you are a diligent manager of money and surround yourself with strong advisors, you may consider a balloon loan.

Our loan was on the seller financed real estate, which he sold to us through this process. So why, you may ask, would you ever do a balloon loan? For us, we wanted to own the building, however the owner didn't want to sell right away. We did note, through conversations, that the seller is planning on retiring to a beach in a few years.

Basically, we agreed to the balloon loan as it allowed the seller to get the remainder of his money right around the time he is probably going to move. For us, we weighed the risks of the balloon loan (i.e. – needing to refinance it in year 5) with the downside of renting the building.

We also utilized a balloon loan in a rather ingenious way, I thought, on a piece of equipment we purchased. After attending a conference / demonstration of some CAD/CAM milling units, we were quickly talked into 'signing on the dotted line' to purchase and finance a unit. Mind you, I could buy a decent home in the Midwest for the cost of one of these units, thus we probably should have given this a bit more thought. Regardless, it served a need and provided financial benefits of not having to pay a lab.

After signing up for the financing through the equipment distributor (higher day 1 rates, but able to be refinanced) – I spoke with my lender and was able to procure a much cheaper interest rate (about half) using a balloon loan. The balloon loan would cover a shorter term and upon the end of my payments, I was going to be required to pay roughly $30k for the remaining balance.

However, as part of the equipment purchase – if we chose to continue buying our consumables / sundry items through the company, they would provide a $10k refund each year for three consecutive years. Thus, I secured a lower rate and had a forced means of 'saving' to pay the $30k at the end of the term. Sometimes creative financing can be beneficial, again please do consult your financial and/or tax advisors and never pursue a balloon loan unless you are disciplined from a financial perspective and have a plan in place to pay off the loan.

Purchase Option:

In case the seller is not willing to sell the building, or if you are nervous about the responsibility / debt associated with buying the real estate, you can consider including a purchase option clause.

A purchase option is the right, but not the responsibility to purchase the property at a specified later date for a pre-specified amount. After the time, say 5 years, elapses, you are then able to call the owner up and tell them you want to exercise the option, you pay them the prespecified amount and go from being a tenant to an owner of your building.

You may have to pay an upfront fee (which can sometimes be rolled into the purchase price) for the right to having this optionality.

Tenant Improvements:

If you have an upcoming lease renewal, or you will be creating a new lease with the seller, you can consider asking for what known as Tenant Improvements. Basically, you're agreeing to sign a lease with the landlord, IF they cover some upfront costs of remodeling, updating, or other needed construction.

My wife attempted to use this approach in her deal as she knew that she needed to update the office in the first year or so. In her case, however, the seller didn't want to pursue this option and opted to offer the sale of the building using seller financing and the balloon loan.

Accounts Receivable:

Buying the accounts receivable is one of the more challenging topics in purchasing a practice. Since most practices are contracted with some number of PPOs, you are likely to see $30k, $50k, or even $100k or more in accounts receivable.

The lower the accounts receivable are, relative to the monthly production, the better the practice is at getting the money from patients and insurance companies.

You, however, need to come up with a way of purchasing the accounts receivable since this is a part of the on-going business operations. We were once told, to simply collect all the money and simply pay out the money to the selling Dr. that they produced, less a 15% collection fee. Thankfully, my wife's mentor (director at her residency program) highly advised against using this approach.

Basically, you would be adding an entirely new dimension to the practice's collection process. You must now positively identify each check coming in as going to Dr. A or Dr. B. Seems easy right – if the check says Dr. A, it goes to them, Dr. B is the same. However, after you purchase the practice you will start receiving checks made out to the old doctor as well as the new doctor with no rhyme or reason. Further, all those AR balances that are pending with insurance are now going to be mailed or electronically credited with your name on it (since you're now credentialed). Literally, your collections person would have to spend significant amounts of time, finding each payments date and compare it to the procedure date and then send over accordingly. Punchline – save yourself the work and do not pursue this method.

The simplest way of transferring AR is to outright buy it, at a discount. The discount is necessary as you're never going to collect 100% of the outstanding balances. Further, what you will find is that the 'marginal' patients who are hit-or-miss on showing up, non-compliant, etc. – if they owe any amount of money, they will use this transition as a way of wiping the slate clean and just disappearing. You're unlikely to collect balances from this population. Hence the reason you must discount the outstanding AR balances; but how much do you discount.

Below is a quick example of a practice which has $50k in outstanding AR. For each time period bucket (age of how long it has been since the procedure was completed/entered), I laid out a few scenarios to consider. In the aggressive scenario, you are paying a lower discount based on the expected collection % for each bucket (basically covers your risk of collecting). This boils down to an 85% Offer Price on AR, which is what you would put into your LOI. The other alternatives shown in this scenario are 75% and 65%. I would probably not take the math literally as you will need to complete your own assessment of risk prior to putting an offer price on the AR in the LOI.

			% Chance of Collecting		
Time	AR	% of Total	Aggressive	Moderate	Conservative
<30	$25,000	50%	95%	90%	85%
30-60	$12,500	25%	85%	75%	65%
60-90	$7,500	15%	75%	55%	35%
90+	$5,000	10%	45%	25%	10%
Total	$50,000	100%	85%	75%	65%

If you do want to adjust some of the % by bucket or by scenario, feel free to visit FirstTimeDentist.com and look for the Practice Evaluation workbook. In it, there will be an "Accounts Receivable" tab with the math already done.

Lastly, always keep the seller's mentality and motivations in mind. The seller has blood, sweat and tears baked-in to those AR balances. The price you place on the AR can carry much more weight because the doctor will be thinking 'you want to pay me 60 cents on the dollar for my last month or two's worth of work?', which is essentially what you're doing.

Balances:

Whenever calculating the amount of AR that you will be buying, you must first back-out the credit balances. Since you're buying an asset (patients owing you money) you must first back-out the money you owe other patients. Thus, the equation would look something like this:

$$\text{AR Purchase Price} = \% \text{ of AR} \times (\text{Total AR} - \text{Credits})$$

However, I would strongly recommend that you set a limit on the total number of credit balances you're willing to purchase. Particularly making sure that credit balances are not over 90 days aged. If you buy those balances, you're also buying a legal obligation to pay them back. Do not inherit the seller's problems or mismanagement (if credit balances are large).

The Seller 'Staying-On':

One of the most underestimated decisions you can make is whether the seller is going to 'stay-on' as an employee, part-owner, associate, advisor, etc. after the transition? In many ways, this is a catch 22. By the seller staying on for a few months after closing, you get the added comfort that you will have some help in navigating the business side of practice ownership. However, there are quite a few downsides to consider here, many of them are personality driven.

If you're considering extending the tenure of the selling doctor, I would closely examine your own and the seller's personalities. The issue is that no matter how many papers you signed, what the new sign says, or how much you borrowed – the dynamic is always going to be to default to the old owner. Employees will do it, patients will do it, and even you will do it.

The question really becomes – how badly do you really need this person? And can the two of you ever really work together? If you have been working with this person for a while, you may have your answer. But if you never had any contact with the seller prior to this engagement – you're taking a risk.

For my wife, she has a very different management style than the selling doctor. He was much more involved in the minutia of the practice, while my wife tends to avoid details and focus on being leadership and her clinical abilities. She prefers to inspire, train, and let people do their jobs as she's not as concerned with how they are getting done, just that they are completed. Neither method is right but had the selling doctor stayed-on as an employee post-close, I can guarantee there would have been fireworks.

While I do not like to proclaim that any method is necessarily the correct way, simply because each situation and individual is unique, I do believe that the seller staying-on post close should be a shorter-term 'gap-fill' vs. a longer-term retirement strategy.

Keep in mind, if you keep them on now you're likely going to be negotiating the seller's salary / production % take-home, benefits, etc. – in addition to all the other typical negotiation points. Negotiating a person's salary, who has been doing this for likely a few decades, can strike a few notes in the heart strings of the seller – as you're essentially telling them how much they are worth vs. how much the more obscure business and patients are worth.

Further, I have heard several horror stories recently which you want to avoid. First, was a dentist who bought a practice from a seller who had a history of doing extremely subpar work. They had the selling doctor 'fill-in' for them after the transition. When the new owner returned, they had patients coming in several months later for a prophy only to find that the 'fillings' done a few months back were extremely questionable and about to fall out. This poor buyer is then forced to 'eat' the costs and tip-toe around the selling Dr's work. This same individual has also recognized what can only be called a systemic failure to deliver the clinical standard of care by the selling Dr. Patients have paid for shotty work for years and now it is all failing. Again, the new owner is having to tread lightly and do a decent amount of free work.

The second horror story I heard was that of an older dentist of a niche practice. The older dentist found and began grooming his successor to move from an associate to an owner and vice versa for the older dentist. After years of working together, training (both clinically and business) and having switched roles – the younger Dr. decided to fire the previous owner (as he was an associate) and asked that he stay off the premises going forward. While I do not know the entire story as to what prompted such a harsh reaction – the punchline is still the same. These two both walked away from the situation feeling slightly.

Again, there is no right way of transitioning a practice. Just make sure that you go in with your eyes wide open. Most business partnerships fail, 50% of marriages end in divorce – and by keeping the seller on, you're essentially entering into the same type of an arrangement.

Retention Bonus:

One neat idea I picked-up during my wife's purchase was the idea of paying the employees a retention bonus (assuming you want them to stay on as employees). While we didn't ask for it, the selling doctor had our best interests in mind and chose to offer to pay employees their standard year-end bonus in the early part of the following year (we closed August 1st), if and only if, they stayed with us through the end of the year. This nearly guaranteed that the employees wouldn't leave as they would be forgoing a few thousand dollars in bonuses if they continued working for only a few more months – enough time for us to somewhat get our feet underneath us.

Again, I'm not suggesting you pursue every one of these options, however if you have any concerns over your employees leaving – this could be an interesting approach to take in the negation process. Logistics of this can get messy, but this is something to consider.

Date of Closing:

Timing is everything. You need to be thoughtful in your due diligence process, asking questions of the broker, seller, etc. Is the doctor wanting to move immediately to Florida? Are they not in a hurry to close? Or are their health concerns that are forcing them to retire early?

You can use the date you are planning to close on as a leverage point. If the doctor is hot to trot on buying a new beach house in the Florida Keys, and he has had little interest in the practice thus far – you could push your date of closing out farther. Doing so, requires that he then respond to your LOI by changing this date. This could prompt a discussion which sounds like this… "Yes, I know selling doctor that you're in a hurry to close, but I'm just not going to be ready for the next few months as I have (XYZ excuse) planned. I suppose I could shorten the timeframe, but hey – about that AR % I offered, what if we moved that down just a bit?".

Remember, it is a give-and-take process. Find out the seller's motivations and limitations and be fluent in your own.

Legal Documents:

While I did mention before that I recommended the seller cover the initial cost of having the lawyers 'draw-up' the paperwork (based on the outcome of the LOI) – you do not necessarily have to pursue this. If you picked up on the seller being overly sensitive to his future legal costs, you could offer to pick this up, in exchange for something else.

Letter of Intent

Often in commercial real estate and other business dealings you will hear the term LOI thrown around early in the purchase process. But what is a LOI?

A Letter of Intent is a semi-formal document used to start the negotiations in a business process. If you've ever purchased a home, it is roughly the same as your purchase price 'offer' made to the seller. The key with an LOI is that it is typically not viewed as a legally binding document (LOI[xxix]). So why should you care about LOIs?

LOIs are actually an extremely beneficial tool that allow you to have an in-depth negotiation with a seller, without the need for updating the pages and pages of legal documents that will surely follow (my wife's purchase required well over 100 pages of dense legal documents).

The LOI is also likely one of the few legal documents that you (the buyer) should be responsible for generating. Make sure you press the seller's attorney to produce most of the legal documents, (they are likely in a substantially better financial position to afford this type of work vs. you who is just starting out), or at least use this as another 'lever'.

Core Components of Your LOI

Ok, now you have the background on the basic negotiation points, here is a list of some items that I would recommend including in an LOI. This list is not all-inclusive, but it should give you basic points and explanations on the sections you're likely to include.

Remember, the sky is the limit, make sure you include anything you want so long as it is a reasonable request from the seller's standpoint.

1. **Purchase Price** – the purchase price is made up of several sub-items and should be broken out with a price for each item. These items will include Equipment, Goodwill, Patient Files, etc. The price associated with each category will be important when you speak with your accountant. This will be equally important for the seller as the more money place in the Goodwill (vs. Fixed Assets like Equipment), the higher the impact both seller's and buyer's taxes.
2. **Non-Compete** – make sure this has a clearly defined time horizon as well as radius/geographic limitations
3. **Accounts Receivable** – you will want to ensure that the amount you'll be paying for outstanding collections is fair, this requires a bit more due diligence as you're very likely to never see some of the prior doctor's patients again, especially the ones who owe a great deal of money or have not made their payments in a timely fashion. Therefore, these balances are worth less (pennies on the dollar) compared to the rest.
4. **Asset Purchase Agreement** – this is a section which can suggest that the largest (and most expensive) part of the negotiation comes from the seller and their attorney
5. **Contingencies** – including financial statement verification, all documents are provided as requested, financing is secured, etc.
6. **Earnest Money** – basically this becomes a non-refundable deposit that, if the LOI is executed, you can lose if you walk away from the practice for any reason not outlined in the contingencies. For this item, I recommend shooting pretty low (start around $1,000). Again, you're likely going to be in a less financially stable situation than the seller, no need to overcommit.
7. **Rent / Occupancy** – Whether you're buying the building for the seller, renting the building from the seller, or renting the building from a separate landlord – you will need to address this in your LOI.
8. **Anything else you want** – remember this is your LOI, this represents your philosophies, goals, limitations, and desires from the practice – make sure you include anything and everything you want – the seller can only say 'no'.

In order to simplify the process even further, I assembled a quick outline of all these points in a form that you can fill-out and hand over to your lawyer (available at FirstTimeDentist.com). The purpose of doing this is to avoid the unnecessary back and forth with your lawyer as you try to construct it, which will hopefully save you money. Remember, they work for you and they will include anything and everything you want included in the LOI.

Keep in mind, continually asking your lawyer for 'sanity checks' on whether this or that is fair or reasonable can be expensive advice. If you have questions that are more business related, try to find a mentor or some other source which is free or cheaper. You can ask what is commonly done, but just remember the lawyer's job is to protect you (his or her client), not create a fair and equitable deal.

Use this template to input all the relevant information and be AS SPECIFIC AS POSSIBLE. Make sure that you include anything and everything in this document (see 'Other Special Requests' at the end of the outline). What you want to avoid is missing any major sticking points early in the process, as they will become larger annoyances towards the end. For instance, if you just assume that the Rembrandt painting is going to stay in the office as it is the focal point of the waiting room – it is going to cause both parties some heartburn when you realize that the seller is taking it home with them.

This type of mishap is likely to occur towards the end of the deal when financing is lined up, vendor relationships are being established, and both parties have already begun to mentally prepare for the transition. You do not want to hurt the relationship (or feelings for that matter) towards the end of the deal, as those are the impressions which will last. Additionally, you do want the seller to continue to be an advocate for you in the community, post-acquisition.

The LOI was one of my greatest failures in the practice purchase process. I kept giving the lawyer information, having them change it, discussing it, refining it, re-reviewing it, etc. Had I just spent the time to assemble all of the below information in a clear, consistent, and concise form – I likely would have saved thousands of dollars. At $300 per hour (or whatever your lawyer's rate is) it doesn't take that many phone calls to start ringing up some serious bills. Further, he delayed the delivery of the LOI (which I did not press him hard enough on) which could have put the deal in jeopardy, had other dentists been actively negotiating as well.

I'm pretty confident in saying that a third to a half of what we spent on legal costs was solely devoted to the LOI. That said, as my lawyer pointed out – if you have a specific and all-inclusive LOI – the rest of the negotiation process should go relatively smoothly, as the LOI becomes the template for the lawyer to draw up all the lengthy paperwork.

A Few Words on Executing the LOI:

As with any negotiation process, there will likely be a few rounds between buyer and seller. In each round, you're hoping to inch closer and closer to landing on an amicable deal for both you and the seller. Work hard to understand the seller's motives

Note the use of the term amicable. I would recommend against 'beating up' the seller on price, or hard/extended negotiations which are difficult, time consuming, and mentally draining for all parties involved. The goal is to come to an amenable price and terms in the shortest timeframe, saving everyone on legal costs.

Keep in mind, that this doctor is likely a member of the community. They may have been practicing here for 10, 15, 20, or even 30 years! You want to get a fair price, of course, but make sure you weigh the opportunity costs of pushing the seller too much – you need him or her on your side after this transaction is completed!

At the end of the day, your goal in this process is to own a successful practice. Let's be honest, you have the ability to make a good deal of money with a practice. Sure, you have to play your cards right, work hard, and strive for excellence, but it is attainable. My advice for settling on a price is to 'not let the dollar fall out of your back pocket as you bend over to pick-up a quarter'. In other words, keep the long-term goals in perspective and do not let a five-thousand dollar now (or whatever the amount is) stop you from realizing your dreams and potentially making hundreds of thousands later.

Financing

Once you and the seller do finally execute the LOI, make sure you get that over to your accountant and your bank quickly. The banker will need to have a copy of this, to allow them to begin drawing up the financial paperwork for the closing.

I will discuss more about the financing process in my last Chapter "Finalizing the Transition". However, for now, just know that the bank is likely to run a credit report, want you to chat on the phone with an underwriter, and that the bank will probably send you an "LOI-Like" offer letter on how much they are willing to lend, over what time period, at what rate ('terms' of the loan).

Make sure that you read everything thoroughly and ask your lender, accountant, or even attorney if you have questions on anything!

Finalizing the Agreements

I chose to break-up the negotiation into two separate sections, the LOI/Offer vs. the Finalizing the Agreements for the simple fact that the majority of your negotiating should be done in the LOI stage. Hopefully by the time you get to the point of finalizing the agreements you have a solid structure for what the transaction is going to look like.

What 'agreements' am I referring to? Well, there's a whole host of documents that you will need to review and sign at your closing. These agreements cover different aspects of the transaction and are all necessary for a complete understanding of how funds will be transferred, what assets go where, and how you will handle/remedy specific issues and situations as they present themselves.

Below is a list of some of the agreements you're likely to run across in the purchase process. Remember, most of these agreements should come from the seller's attorney (unless you want to use this as a bargaining chip). Additionally, not every deal will require each agreement and this is not a comprehensive list of all the agreements you may encounter.

Legal Agreements for Practice Purchase:

1. **Asset Purchase Agreement:** This is the primary agreement which will detail the litany of assets that will be transferred during the sale. Additionally, it covers operational components such as re-work, employees, and utility transfers.
2. **Affidavit of Solvency and Asset Ownership** - This is document may or may not be necessary (ask your lawyer) as it helps to establish that the seller of the practice is the true owner of the practice and that they do not have any outstanding financial issues.
3. **Real Estate Purchase Agreement** - Pretty self-explanatory agreement, outlines the details of the transfer of the property (purchase price, contingencies, etc.).
4. **Promissory Note** - Similar to what you may have signed for your student loans, a promissory note is straight-forward, it basically says that you promise to pay the money you're being loaned back to the lender and contains some basic information on the loan. This would likely come from the bank, or the seller if seller-financed.
5. **Mortgage** - The mortgage works in conjunction with your promissory note, as a way of detailing some of the requirements of the lender, for their security (i.e. – maintenance of property, paying real estate taxes, insurance requirements, eminent domain, etc.).
6. **Warranty (or other) Deed** - This is the official transfer of property which will need to be recorded with local agencies. Read carefully and pay

attention to the details when transferring the title to avoid complicated issues later. When we were closing on my wife's practice, I read over the deed and noticed a very small error/omission. I questioned whether it even mattered and the title agency didn't even hesitate to go correct the issue and reprint the deed – they want it done correctly too!

7. **Bill of Sale** - At the end of the day, this is really the 'official' document which shows that the practice has been transferred from Doctor A to Doctor B. It is synonymous to the relationship between the Warranty Deed and the Real Estate Purchase Agreement.
8. **Closing Statement** - Not so much of a legal statement, more of a detailed account of how escrow funds, funds used to purchase the practice, and broker commissions are paid. This might not be available until you close, if you are buying the AR (calculated as of close that day/day before).
9. **Rental Agreement** - If you are unable or unwilling to buy the building you will need to secure a commercial lease agreement with the landlord who can either be the seller or some other entity. Please, I stress PLEASE, do not ever sign a lease with a landlord without seeking legal guidance. Laws protect residential renters from being unfairly taken advantage of by savvy landlords. However, there are no such restrictions in the commercial realm.

In finance and business, we often say "Caveat Emptor" which is Latin saying used in business meaning "Buyer Beware". Legally, commercial businesses tend to have much lower amounts of protection for the owner. It is the assumption of government and the judicial system that being in businesses automatically makes you savvy in business OR at least savvy enough to solicit professional help.

Commercial leases can be filled with landmines, sneaky tricks, etc. Do not get sucked into a bad lease by not getting help or not getting the right help (make sure your lawyer regularly looks at leases).

Also, if you are planning on owning the building, ask your lawyer about the option of holding the real estate in a separate entity (LLC) than your dental practice. You can then have a commercial lease between the entities to add an additional layer of legal (and financial) protections. Do consult your lawyer on whether this is the best strategy and their thoughts on avoiding a situation where you 'piece the corporate veil'.

Next Steps

After I described to my wife all the documents I had received, she was surprised to learn that I wanted her to read them. She kept asking 'Why do I need to read them if I have a lawyer, isn't that what we pay him for?'.

Yes, you will pay your lawyer quite a bit of money to read these agreements and advise you of the pitfalls, if any. However, as I discussed with my wife, the lawyer is responsible for telling you the pros and cons of what you're getting into, not how to fulfil the agreement.

For example, we have a mortgage with the selling doctor. Each month, I'm required to pay him principal + interest on the building loan. My lawyer agreed that the mortgage seemed standard and was worth signing. However, my lawyer is not in charge of making sure I mail the check to the seller each month, I am.

The same goes for the Asset Purchase Agreement, or any of the other agreements you will sign in this process. You need to make sure that you fully understand what is written on each and every page you will receive. Fun fact, I counted and the number of pages my wife and I had to review was in excess of 100 pages. Yes, that's 100 pages of dense legalese that your gut will likely want to avoid reading. Here are a few quick steps to follow to make the process a bit easier:

Do not do it all in one session: My wife may have procrastinated this task just a bit. Then, late on a Thursday night (2 days before our wedding) the broker informed me that the seller's attorney was (unexpectedly) going on a 2-week vacation and was hoping to read our revisions before she left. This caused quite a bit of unnecessary stress before our 'big day'. Point is, this material is dense and difficult, set a goal to read and fully understand one agreement per day. You may even want to re-read each before contacting your lawyer for comments/questions. Second learning point – make sure you know the related party's (lawyers, sellers, brokers, etc.) vacation schedule.

Skim the legalese, focus on the content: You will read a lot of stuff that sounds like "Pursuant to the decree handed out on the fifth day of June (June 5) of the year of our Lord 2017, in section 4.1.03c of the Ohio Revised Code...". While I may have embellished a bit here, the point remains the same focus on the sections that directly pertain to your day-to-day and skim the rest.

...But read it all: While I suggest skimming through the legalese that does not mean you do not read each document in its entirety – you must know what you're signing as you are in charge of 'making it happen.'

Go back to D-School: My wife talks fondly about her day's studying pharmacy back in D-School. Actually, I'm just kidding - to this day, watch her get a cold chill as she walks into a Panera (her favorite studying spot where she would construct a war room like gathering of colored pens, highlighters, notes, and textbooks). My point is this – get these same pens, highlighters, and notebooks ready and red-line the hell of those documents. Everything you do not understand is in yellow, everything you want to remove in red, and everything you want to add in blue. The color scheme doesn't really matter, so much as the notes and the ongoing learning involved with these documents.

Setup a call with your lawyer: notating the agreements and sending them back to your lawyer is not enough. Schedule a follow-up meeting with him or her to review, in great and painful detail, each question you have on each page of the agreements. This is necessary for you to be a fully informed owner and might be something you consider doing 'in-person'.

Final Iterations

As you are reviewing the documents, your lawyer should simultaneously be reviewing them so that they can provide their input. You will probably go through a few document revisions whereby your lawyer sends you a list of proposed changes, you approve, and then their sent over to the seller's lawyer.

On the seller's side, they will be taking the same approach – reading your updated documents, lawyer providing input, suggesting changes, and then sending them back to you for review. This can be a very tedious segment in the process of buying a practice. By now, you have probably reached a consensus on the sale price, the cost of AR, and a host of other points. Yet you find yourself negotiating on some finer points in the deal or legal language.

For instance, my lawyer suggested removing a clause (which is usually standard in mortgages, I was told) that waives the buyer's rights to a trial, should we have gone into default on the mortgage for the building. While this was standard, the lawyer said that he represented me and my interests only and suggested striking that from the contract. We sent a revised version to the seller and their attorney did not have a problem with most changes, but then added that clause back into the contract.

We could have gone back-and-forth negotiating hard to get this portion of the mortgage removed, however it was more-or-less a 'bonus' for us all along. We did not bother trying to remove the cause on the second 'turn' of the documents.

Point is, similar to negotiating the price of the deal – do not let the entire thing fall apart because of some of the finer points in the deal. While it is certainly more of an art than a science, you want to make sure that you know when to fight for a clause (or removal) and when to just weigh and accept the risks.

Recap

Some people love negotiating. The thrill of the chase. The hard-nosed attitude. Some people even enjoy trying to put the screws to the seller as much as possible.

Remember as you go through this process that you are attempting to put a price on the seller's life's work. You have probably heard the term 'it's strictly business' and while that is true in many respects. You mustn't forget the genuinely personal aspect of this process. If you approach negotiations as simply a dance in which both individuals are moving in the same direction with some give-and-take, you are much more likely to end in a mutually beneficial position.

At the end of the day, you are always going to look back and question – did I pay too much? Should I have asked for this or that? Etc. I once heard that the fairest transactions are ones where neither the seller nor the buyer walks away feeling like they got everything in which they wanted. And that's OK!

Remember that the long-term goal is for you to be a practice owner. While I certainly do not want you to overpay for a practice, in 10 or 15 years – an extra $5,000 or even $10,000 is really not going to make or break you. Some people may take this as too lassie faire of an attitude but remember how all this started was your vison. A vision without action is just a dream that never comes to reality. You're better to pursue a vision and make some mistakes along the way then to not pursue the vision and have a void or regret in life.

Happy negotiating!

CHAPTER 7: CLOSING

"If you can't fly then run, if you can't run then walk, if you can't walk then crawl, but whatever you do you have to keep moving forward." -Martin Luther King Jr.

You made it! You are finally at the stage where you are starting to think – 'this really is going to happen!'. In this last Chapter of this book, I would like to focus on making sure that you have a clear plan for what closing day is going to look like, in addition to explaining all the necessary steps leading up to closing.

I have assembled a detailed checklist of all the items that will need completed prior to your closing day. You can find the checklist/time-line at FirstTimeDentist.com. This checklist will provide you quick reminders, while the remaining part of this Chapter we be more of an expose on the specific details for each item on the checklist.

You are about to enter a world of paperwork. From vendor transfer forms, new bank account information to credentialing and government registrations - the amount of paperwork will be intimidating. That's where I come in, however. I hope to make this process as seamless as possible and provide you with an organized approach and a detailed understanding.

One of your best assets in this section is going to be what I call the 'Practice Cheat Sheet'. I will provide you more information later, but just knows that without this quick reference tool, there is NO way that I could have ever made it through the process myself. Take my advice, use the provided template (or make your own) and save yourself the hassle of looking for information later, as you will inevitably need every piece of confidential personal and professional information for a multitude of reasons.

Pre-Closing Checklist

Much of the content in the next two sections of this Chapter is going to be punch-list items that need completed. Below is a high-level overview of each items in a semi-sequential order. I say 'semi-sequential' as every scenario will be different but should follow the same general pattern. I will go through, in much greater detail, the individual items in the following sections.

Pre-Closing Checklist:
1. Finalize Dates and Times
2. Patient Letters
3. Building Inspection
4. Credentialing Process
5. Finalize Insurance
6. Finalize Lending
7. Website Transition
8. Setup Payroll
9. Bank Accounts
10. Accounting
11. Branding
12. Marketing
13. Items to Purchase
14. Employees / Human Resources

Item 1: Finalize Dates and Times

If you haven't already, formally set the closing date. Attempt to plan the closing to be on a Thursday at the end of a month (allows for utilities to be transferred on Friday, a workday).

I would make sure that you formally request the seller to be available (in-office) the day after the closing. This allows you to ask any last questions. To have them work with you to ensure vendors have transferred, etc.

Establish the date in which employees will be told (like 1-2 weeks prior to closing) about the up-coming transaction.

Setup a time with the Doctor (a day or so after the employees are told) to visit the office and do a 'meet and greet' with the staff. Consider bringing them some light snacks or refreshments, if done after a day of work.

Consider doing a week of 'shadowing' prior to close. This is in-office learning whereby you sit and watch the interactions between the Dr. and patients, employees and patients, and between employees. Take a small notebook and jot down ideas on how to improve things in the long-haul (do not make changes day 1).

If you do choose to pursue the week of shadowing – I would also recommend that you take each employee out to lunch during that week, on your dime, a place of their choosing, and only one at a time. More on this later in the 'Employees' Section.

Item 2: Patient Letters

As part of the transition, the seller will need to write a letter to each patient and send them (on their dime) to officially announce the transition. You should include a short bio in the letter and give your approval over its content, prior to them being sent out.

It is also recommended that you take a nice photo with you and the seller prior to closing and include that in the letter. Ensure these are approved ahead of time, so as not to back the seller in the corner when they are trying to get 1,000's of letters printed.

Item 3: Building Inspection

If you are purchasing the building, this would be the time to hire a Commercial Property Inspector (not residential) to walk through the building. Doing so can provide peace of mind, but also give you a short-list of items that need fixed. Make sure you plan this after-hours and get the full approval and cooperation of the seller.

Item 4: Begin Credentialing Process

One of the biggest tasks is dependent on how many insurance providers the Dr. is currently 'credentialed' with (i.e. – 'in-network'). Essentially, you need to contact each insurance company and find out the process of transferring credentialing status from the seller to you.

To complete the myriad of forms, I would recommend starting to collect all the possible information you will need (Driver's License, SSN #, TIN # of new business, NPI #, DEA #, Address/Dates of your collegiate school history, etc.) – Practice 'Cheat-Sheet'.

Next, get a written list of every insurance company you want to be 'in-network' with, along with the level(s) in which they are currently credentialed (for instance you can be part of the XYZ 300, 400, or 500 network).

The forms they request you submit can be daunting. My biggest piece of advice is to make copies of these forms before returning. We had to get 're-credentialed' 2 years after owning, I can't tell you how great it would have been to have a copy of the original form so that I could reference it and not have to look up all the data.

If you plan to be credentialed with any government programs (i.e. – Medicaid) you need to start this process as soon as possible. As is dealing with any government agency – there is quite a bit of paperwork and lead time needed (could be months!).

Item 5: Insurance Agent

If you haven't already found an insurance agent (refer back to Chapter 2 – Building Your Team) make sure you find someone soon. Prior to closing you should have in-place or ready to go the following types of insurance:

1. Malpractice
2. General Business Liabilities (Property & Casualty)
3. Employees (Property & Casualty)
4. Data Security (Property & Casualty)
5. Disability / Overhead
6. Life
7. Umbrella Policy

Keep in mind, you will likely need proof of insurance for your lender so the sooner you get this ready, the better. That said, for the last 3 listed (Disability / Overhead, Life, and Umbrella) these are items which either take longer to procure or you may need to actually own the practice. So, start working on them quickly, but do not expect to have them in place by closing.

Item 6: Finalize Lending

You need to be in 'lock-step' with your lender throughout the latter half of the process. You will likely get lots of e-mails during the underwriting process asking you to send paperwork, submit forms, documentation, or other information. Do it as expediently as possible.

You will likely need to meet with an underwriter so that they can ask you about your experience (clinically and business) as well as your plans for the future. Certainly, being honest in this process is necessary. But do not be afraid to mention seemingly esoteric facts, if they support your business or clinical aptitude. Did you take extra CE in residency? What practice management courses or books have you read (if any) - mention them! Helped your dad do books at his pet store growing up? That's business experience!

If the lender isn't already reaching out to you on a regular basis, I would make sure you have at least a once / week touchpoint with them to ensure that everything is on-track.

Item 7: Website Transition

In an ideal world, you would have a web-site up-and-running day 1 of you walking into your practice. It would be complete with all the bells-and-whistles imaginable allowing for a seamless transition from the old Dr. In reality, developing a website that is to your liking is a long-haul process and not something that will be complete overnight.

My advice is to first plan on having the selling Dr. post an announcement on their website (complete with a link to the patient letter) the day after closing. Their site should stay up and active (or automatically re-direct to your site) for several months.

Second, for the over-achiever, I would actually start a website prior to owning. I think the important thing here is to secure the domain name that you desire. The content, layout, hosting, etc. can always be moved, transferred, and updated. In my opinion, you're better off having a website with OK content, then you are to have no website at all.

There are a host of websites available offering pre-built/drag-and-drop options (think WIX.com) which will allow you to cheaply get something up and running.

Remember that building a business that is 'to your liking' is a lifetime pursuit, not something that can be accomplished overnight.

Item 8: Payroll Vendor

Establishing a relationship with the payroll vendor early in the process is ideal. Payroll, as you may expect, is not something that you can mess around with. It must be on-time, accurate, and easy to use for you.

There are many reputable companies (ADP, Paychex, QuickBooks) which offer payroll services. You can also check with your accountant to see if they offer payroll services.

A learning points we had was that because the owner of my wife's practice was doing payroll themselves, they could process payroll on a Wednesday and pay on a Thursday. Once we got involved with a payroll company (and since we were still getting a few paper checks) we actually found out that the days required for the new payroll schedule would cause the employees to basically have a one-week gap in pay, while the old system phased out and the new one started booking hours. Give your employees notice here, remember this is their livelihoods and should be taken seriously.

That said, one thing to consider is moving to a 2x / month paycheck (vs. every other week). While this may seem inconsequential at first, it actually causes a few headaches down the road. The primary issue is that being paid every other week (known as Bi-weekly) requires that you cut 28 paychecks throughout the year. Thus, there will always be 2 months with 3 paychecks.

This can cause a bit of a strain on financials during these 3-check months. However, by doing 2x / month (say 1-15th pay period, pay on the 20th and 15th – 30th / 31st, pay on the 5th) you can avoid these months and spread out those two checks to the other 26 checks during the year. Additionally, this has a 'soft' benefit of providing you more accurate intra-month reporting, if and when you ever start working with a consultant or tracking your performance through more powerful management software and reporting tools.

I would also make sure you have a system setup with the vendor where by 'ticklers' or 'reminder' notices, e-mails, calls, are sent out. It could take a few months before you get into the payroll rhythm. This applies to situations whereby you are paying every-other-week (recommended). If the current Dr. is paying weekly, it is going to be a harder message to deliver to the employees, however the Dr. is quite literally doubling their payroll expense.

In general, you will probably pay $10-$25 / employee / paycheck. There are also fees for W2s at the end of the year, if you opt for full-service payroll (recommended).

Item 9: Open Bank Account

You will want to have a business banking relationship established prior to closing. This will allow you to easily deposit the initial working capital, start running expenses through the business, as well as establish direct deposit connections for insurance companies, merchant services (credit card payments) and auto-deductions for utilities.

Products you will need include a basic Checking and Savings account, a Credit Card, a Line of Credit (if the bank is not providing working capital), and a merchant services relationship for credit card processing. Do ensure that your credit card processing unit is installed / tested prior to your first day.

In terms of 'good practices' it is always good to make sure that your bank statements are delivered and opened by you. Doing so allows for you to be the first person to see and hold the statement, intercepting the chances of fraud. This risk is obviously lessened in today's digital age, when you can access easily online or over your phone. However, for this reason, I would recommend that all credit card statements, bank statements, or other sensitive financial information be addressed to your personal residence and not the business.

I would order two sets of paper checks / checkbooks – one for home and one for your office.

Assuming you are buying the AR outright - make sure that you also let the bank know that you will be depositing checks in both the name of your business as well as the prior doctor's. They should be able to notate on the account, though you may have to show some documentation.

Item 10: Accounting

Decide whether you want to manage your own bookkeeping (i.e. – working in QuickBooks) or if you want your accountant to do so. Do note, if you're completely new to QuickBooks and/or have little financial background – I would kick this over to the accountant. I have a degree in finance and eventually got sick of the accounting piece and have our accountant handle ours now.

If you are choosing to do it yourself, you should still send the list of the initial expenses you have personally incurred to your accountant. They can take this information and begin setting up your 'chart of accounts' which is basically your income/expenses categories you will see on you monthly reports. They can then return a QuickBooks file (or whatever accounting software you chose) allowing you to begin managing your finances.

If you are not choosing to do it yourself, it is still good to send the list of expenses and have the accountant get your accounting system setup. I would also recommend meeting with them and finding out the process by which they will manage your books.
1. What receipts / statements do they need? When?
2. What reports will you receive from them? When?
3. Other information they will need?

Item 11: Branding

Since you are starting a business, you will need to develop some 'brand assets' to be used on business cards, letter heads, mailings, etc.

I would start by designing a basic logo with an appropriate font, possibly a slogan to include with your logo – you can always improve it later!

To do so, check out 99designs.com, Fiverr or other Elance, or other online freelancing sites. This website offers, for a very reasonable price, the ability to submit a request to a network of 100's or 1,000's of designers. They will take what you request and draw up some prototypes. The logo you like the most can be fine-tuned and then sent to you digitally (and you get the full design copyright).

I would also consider finding a local printer or Vistaprint and buy the following:
1. Letterheads for billing or other official letters
2. Business cards with appointment reminders on back (start with 1,000)
3. Checks with business name / account on them (if your bank doesn't give you a starter kit)
4. Pre-printed envelopes / labels, or an ink stamp with the businesses address on it
5. 'For deposit only' stamp for any checks you receive

Item 12: Marketing Strategy

Similar to the website transition discussed above, I would not recommend spending too much time analyzing each marketing strategy that the selling Dr. currently has implemented and optimizing your marketing spend.

In general, this is a time of 'make it work' vs. 'make it perfect'. Your goal should be to complete a quick survey of the marketing efforts taken on by the current Dr. and transition thoughts to supporting you and your future practice.

If the selling Dr. has any print advertising, they may have actually pre-paid for these ads, so you may be able to send the company your information and brand items in an effort to swap out the selling Dr.'s program for yours.

At a minimum, however, you should quickly assemble a Facebook page and have at the ready an announcement to send out from the selling Dr.'s profile and/or your own to generate some buzz and notify the community.

Item 13: Items to Purchase

Prior to closing, make sure you have a list of any additional office items you need to buy or order prior to closing. These items may include computers, artwork, décor, or other items in which the seller has specifically requested to take with them

Additionally, after completing your equipment checklist in Chapter 5, you may have some additional clinical instruments or equipment to order prior to day 1 in the office.

Item 14: Employees / Human Resources

Employees are an important part of your day. Possibly the most important part of your day, in fact. Patients will quickly pick-up on the level of excitement, job satisfaction, and generally happiness (or lack-thereof) without much effort. Thus, it is crucial that you get off to a good start with your employees. I am going so suggest several ideas to help you in this transitional period. Obviously, you do not have to follow these ideas verbatim, but they should spark at least a thought or two on how to engage and win-over employees in this early phase.

Setting the Stage

One of the biggest concerns with you taking over the helm, is change. Change can come in many forms, whether its new responsibilities, different expectations, wages, benefits, or even whether you keep your job or not. In order to instill some confidence, I would specifically talk with the employees and state that you are making the strategic decision to make as few changes as possible for the first 3-6 months (within reason). This shows that you are committed to first learning how they do business today, allowing you time to game-plan on what can be improved.

Additionally, you need to make them feel important (because they are!) by listening to them and any suggestions they have. As I discussed in the Pre-Closing Checklist section – I would recommend taking each employee to lunch during the week you are shadowing. Make sure they chose the place (within reason or from a short-list of locales). You want this meeting to be very informal learning session for you. First and foremost, you want to learn about each person – where did they grow up? Where do they live? Are they married? Kids? Hobbies? Get to know them personally first, then transition the discussion towards their thoughts on how the practice is run and how it can be improved. Let them know that you took them to lunch in order to provide them an opportunity to say anything they want, good or bad, about the practice, owner, employees, processes, etc. Depending on the personality type, it may be easier to get this information out of people in this type of an environment, than a weekly team meeting.

Lastly, make sure you pay for the meal, without hesitation. Show the employees that you are thankful for them and that you look forward to working with them, by being their host.

Pay and Job Security

In the process of buying a practice, the old owner will usually terminate the employee's jobs and then you are essentially 'rehiring' them. In order to rehire them, you will want to make sure the following paperwork is completed for each employee:

1. IRS Form W-4
2. State Tax Forms
3. Local Tax Forms
4. Department of Homeland Security
5. Payroll Vendor's form (Direct Deposits, Employee Information, etc.)

Remember, that you surveyed their salaries back in Chapter 5, in order to understand if anyone was over/under-paid. If you did in fact determine that someone is over-paid and you want to 'correct' that, you have the right to change their pay up or down. However, it should be quite apparent that taking someone's pay down (especially a tenured individual) is likely to cause them to leave. This can be good or bad.

If you already have some issues with how the person conducts themselves, as you sometimes find very dominating personalities from office managers or otherwise who have been at a practice for a very long time, you may think about trying to 'oust' them early. Firing employees, once hired, can be a more involved process. The employee can file for unemployment, requiring more paperwork and reporting from you, and you can always run the risk of legal actions for unfair termination by the employee. So, think long and hard about hiring any of these employees, if you are not fond of them.

Beyond that, there is certainly risks associated with not hiring on any of the employees that worked for the previous doctor. In that scenario, you are immediately thrust into finding a replacement by placing ads, interviewing, and ensuring they will fit in with the rest of the team. This can be an unnecessary amount of stress when you are just starting out so think long and hard about your next steps here.

That said, if you do decide that keeping the employees is the most logic approach, tell them! Make sure you explicitly say, I plan on hiring all of you onto my new practice. Remember, they are moms and dads who have families with children to feed and bills to pay. When my wife came in to meet the team when they were first told about the practice being sold, she said you could just see the fear in the eyes of some of them. They were quite concerned about whether they would have a job in a few weeks or not. Settle those fears, when able.

Benefits

The benefits that the selling doctor offers are just that – his or her benefits, not yours. I would spend to educate the employees that while you may be keeping things 'the same' for the first few months, there may be changes eventually. Take the time to craft a 1-page handout of the benefits you offer to employees. Think about it as if you were interviewing an employee that you really liked. You would want to hand them something in which you have a great deal of price. You want to be a good employer, as that attracts good employees.

All that said, I would caution against trying to replicate any type of retirement plan that is in place for employees, at least initially. The issue here is that you have not experience what a typical month, or year looks like (financially) when you are the owner. Keep in mind the financials from the seller are likely going to be biased upwards (i.e. – more profitable) as the seller will almost certainly have less debt than what you're about to borrow. Additionally, retirement plans require a great deal of setup (~2-hour initial call covering extremely detailed items, paperwork, and lots of follow-ups). Retirement plans also require additional work to get payroll possessing successfully integrated with your current payroll provider.

My advice is to be transparent with employees, stating that you would like to reinstate the plan, at some point, but are currently choosing to abandon retirement savings until you can gain a better picture of the financial situation. As always, do not even think to attempt this on your own. Chat with your accountant, or better yet, your financial advisor for more details on how/when to implement a plan.

Closing Day – What to Expect

The day of your closing, finally! All the work you have done for the past few months all comes to a head at this crescendo of the practice purchase process. While nothing in this section will probably come as a shock to you, I did want to present a start-to-finish view of what closing day will look like and things you need to keep in mind.

Who Will be Present:
1. Seller(s)
2. Seller's Broker
3. Your Broker (if you have one)
4. Notary (Broker should have this certification)
5. You / Significant Other
6. Banker / Lender (Optional)

I do not think that it is necessary to bring your attorney, accountant as every agreement should have been thoroughly vetted by this point. You may need your banker to be present (if they so choose) to complete the transfer of funds.

Possible Closing Time-Line:
- **30 Minutes** – Greetings, getting organized
- **15 Minutes** – finalizing AR purchase amount (if buying outright) – requires taking the most recent AR report, adjusting for 'credit' balances (monies owed to patients) and then applying a % ratio to the outstanding amount.
- **45 Minutes** – sign paperwork, lots of it. You will probably need to sign/initial 2-3 copies of each document (one for buyer, seller, and either broker or attorney).
- **1-2 Hours** – travel to title agency and complete the transfer of the building (if purchasing)
- **1-2 Hours** – I would recommend going out to eat with all those who were at the closing. This is a monumental change for both you and the selling Doctor – now celebrate! Make friends with the selling Doctor as much as possible, you never know when you may need them in the future.

CHAPTER 8: POST CLOSING

"A hero is no braver than the ordinary man, but he is braver five minutes longer" – Ralph Waldo Emerson

Congratulations. If you have completed the closing step, you have accomplished what few have done in life, to buy a business! This is a monumental step in your goal towards personal and professional success. I can assure you that someday you will lookback at this experience with a sentimental affection as having pursued the path of ownership will change the direction of your life.

Now that the legal and lending stuff has been handled, make sure that you immediately start taking steps towards ensure your first week (and subsequent weeks) get off to a great start. Below is a checklist of items that I would recommend working through. Again, this is not meant to be a fully applicable or all-inclusive list but do consider each item and how it pertains to your individual situation.

Post-Closing Checklist:
1. Transfer Utilities
2. Security and Access
3. Bank Account / Payments
4. Procedures and Your First Week
5. Register / Update Dental Licensures
6. Confirm Completion of Credentialing
7. List out Short-Term Goals
8. Thank You's

Item 1: Transfer Utilities

Utilities can be a notoriously tricky endeavor. Ensuring that you have the seller's devoted attention the day after closing allows you to focus on transferring all utilities, which may require getting account numbers, verification of identities, or other requirements. Make sure you have your cheat sheet ready, along with a copy of the bill of sale and your checkbook.

Utilities to transfer include:
1. Water
2. Gas
3. Electric
4. Cable
5. Phone
6. Internet
7. Others

Item 2: Security and Access

Can you think of a worse scenario – coming into work on your first day and being locked out of the building because you forgot to get the security code? What about not being able to access software or a website which is used on a daily basis at the office? This step should help you avoid those pitfalls by making sure all necessary passwords, codes, pins, keys, etc. have been transferred to you:

1. Keys to practice
2. Security system code
3. Profile setup or password for practice management software
4. WiFi Password(s)
5. Additional profiles / passwords for all software used in office:
    -Payroll services / time management software?
    -Appointment Confirmation Software?
    -Vendor / ordering websites?
    -Insurance websites?

Item 3: Bank Account / Payments

After all this work, it would be a shame to not have any cash flow in your practice for the first week. I read once about someone who had not transferred over the account properly with their insurance companies and ended up having to wait a week or so until they could get the EFTs (electronic funds transfer) setup correctly. The lesson is to make sure that you work with your credentialed insurance companies and your billing department to ensure that there is no disruption in payments.

Additionally, I would make a phone call or stop into your bank and speak with your business banker about cashing any checks in the previous owner's name. Assuming that you're buying the AR, you are entitled to any and all monies owed to the prior doctor.

While less and less checks are being written these days with the access to digital tools, you may be surprised just how many checks will be written to you for payment. Further, you will also be surprised on the wide array of what people will write in for the Payee on the checks ("Dr. Seller", "Dr. Seller LLC", "Dr. Buyer", "Dr. Buyer and Dr. Seller", etc.).

You want to talk with your banker and make sure that any checks made out to the previous owner for provided dental services, can be cashed / deposited against your account. They may require proof of sale or a purchase agreement to do so.

Item 4: Procedures and Your First Week

Most offices have some set procedures – whether explicitly documented (ideal) or in everyone's heads (most common). Regardless, you want to understand those procedures and Systems as much as possible and get a copy of any and all documents that exist.

Focus on your first week and walk through all the motions, asking yourself 'what do I need to know about how this office runs to make this a successful week?' Do not focus on month-end or year-end closing of the books or other esoteric / uncommon occurrences. Just focus on the here and now. If you did not have a chance to shadow or mystery shop the office, consider bringing in your team and doing some role playing and/or further discussion on tasks and who owns each. The more prepared you are for Day/Week 1, the less stress you're likely to undergo.

More tactically, here are a few additional items to request from the Dr:
1. Demonstration of the opening /closing procedures for the office each day.
2. Demonstration of 'key' reports and process of pulling out of practice management software.
3. Upcoming vacation schedule for employees / closed office days.
4. Walk-through of your first weeks' worth of patients (if Seller is walking away day 1).

Item 5: Register / Update all Dental Licensures

You should also check to ensure the following licensures are updated with your most current information:
1. NPI (National Provider Identifier[xxx])
2. DEA # (Drug Enforcement Administration[xxxi])
3. State Board
4. X-Ray / Radiation

I would also work with your dental software provider to make sure doctor names and/or other information can be updated. You want to avoid having the selling doctor's name on billing statements or receipts being sent out on Monday.

Item 6: List Out Goals for 1st Year:

This doesn't have to be a huge task, but I think it is important to list out 3-5 goals for yourself over the coming months. The goals should be simple, attainable, but focused on surviving your first week.

Here are a few examples to consider:

- **Week 1:** Make a positive impact on one patient
- **Month 1:** Gain a better understanding of how employees work together
- **Month 3:** Begin to document short-comings
- **Month 6**: Finalize document on short-comings, consider how to address
- **Month 12:** Celebrate first year of practice, hold off-site team meeting to discuss 2nd year and ideas on short-comings

Item 7: Confirm Completion of Credentialing:

Continual follow-up with Insurance companies / PPOs that you may be participating with is essential – as they are not very good at returning calls or responding to e-mails. Keep in mind, that even if you are not credentialed on the first day, you should still be able to submit claims, the insurance company is just going to recognize this as an 'Out of Network' Provider.

This is probably not the best experience for the patient as it could cost them more, but the impacts are limited to the time it takes for you to get the stamp of approval.

Item #8: Thank You's

At the conclusion of the first week, month, or some other anniversary (preferably in first 2-3 months) - I would recommend doing something special for your employees. Remember, they will be under additional stress as well for the first few months. It is not unusual to hear about employees working at an office for 10, 15, or even 20+ years, suddenly a new doctor comes in with different preferences, ideas and training. You do not have to spend a significant amount of money on your employees, just a handwritten card with a small gift (restaurant gift card, bottle of wine, flowers, candy, etc.).

Send these items to the employee's home to allow the gift to feel very personal and thoughtful. Your goal here is to build a relationship with employees. Small gifts with personalized notes can go a long way in saying 'I appreciate you and working hard through this transitional time period.'

How to Survive Your First Week

Please, watch this video and take to heart the excitement and emotion that Will Smith discusses in his own experiences with Sky Diving. You will probably have points of maximum fear during procedures, facing employee issues, patient issues, etc. The whole point is once you push past that fear, past that point of telling yourself that 'you can't' and move towards 'how can I?' – that is the inflection point that matters.

You will face challenges, lots of them in this process. Your goal for the first week is to do nothing more than survive the first week. Do not try to optimize, change, improve, or otherwise disturb the flow of the office. Your goal is simply to 'get by' from a management perspective. Why, you may ask, is a self-proclaimed 'businessman' telling you to avoid the business side of the equation as much as possible? Unlike other industries, you are part CEO, accountant, front office manager, salesperson, and manufacturer. Even if you have an office manager, it is still your business and you need to be involved in all aspects of your business – eventually.

For today, for just the first week – enjoy your accomplishment and focus on getting to know the patients, providing excellent clinical care, and learning how your employees work. The time for change will come but resist the urge at this stage.

Living Life and Improving Your Practice

While it may sound counter-intuitive to so quickly recommend taking a vacation after having just closed on your practice, it is unbelievably important. Please ensure that you have a vacation schedule in the first 6-12 months after closing. You need time away to decompress, reenergize and create a plan of how to transform the practice and make it your own in the coming years.

No matter how closely aligned the practice is to your original goals, there is always going to be a gap between what you have and what you want. While that gap, hopefully, shrinks over time – your goal as a leader is to always word on skills needed to facilitate change in your practice.

Being a leader is crucial in dentistry. Micro-managing your team is neither productive nor feasible – thus breeding a collaborative and independent team is going to be a necessary feature of your plan. Beyond having a morning meeting / huddle to discuss the patients of the day, I would also recommend you consider facilitating an even high degree of communication. When I mean high, I mean weekly 1-2-hour meetings to discuss necessary topics. I watched my wife, who is practice is operating above her capacity (booking prophy's for 8 to 9 months out) take this approach and the results have been astounding.

At the advice of her business coach – she literally closes the practice for an hour and then rolls into lunch each Wednesday. Everyone is required to be in attendance for these meetings (even the part-time employees not working that day). She uses the time to talk about successes, failures, and where she wants to go with the practice. She started a book club with her team and they discuss how to apply the book's lessons to the personal and professional lives. I have watched as her team has transformed from a robot mindset, to independent free-thinkers.

All this, because they took the time to sit and talk each week. Did it cost her/us money due to lost production, covering the costs of lunch and the additional paid lunch they get? Yes, in the short-term it did probably cost us more. However, the long-term benefits are already being realized, less than 1 year since she started this protocol. I urge you to be open minded and consider this and other off-site team events which allow for the free exchange of ideas and concerns – without the distraction of phone calls and patients in the waiting room.

Conclusion

Unlike the rest of the practice purchase process, the process of physically (and legally) closing is actually one of the easier portions. Mostly this section is about using the provided checklist (or making your own) and following it within the correct timeframe.

You will find as you go through the process of becoming a business owner, that checklists are your friend. You need them to get through each of your procedures, challenges, and days. Checklists become a great way of capturing long-term goals, changes you would like to make in the practice (but aren't going to make immediately) or equipment to buy.

There are many quotes to pull from (most over-used) but just know that this entire process of advancing your career is a process. Notate where you can improve and work on getting there, but do not expect any change will bring immediate gratification. It will take 5-10 years to get the practice operating the way you want, patience is a virtue.

Congratulations on taking the first step towards practice ownership. You truly are making one of the best decisions in your life and I hope that the outcome exceeds your expectations and provides you with a sense of fulfillment that is unmatched until this point in your life. I urge you to always strive for excellence, never comprise your authenticity, and "provide the same care to your patients as you would if it was [your] own grandmother sitting in your chair" (quote from my wife).

Adam Heim

FINAL THOUGHTS

Every man's life ends the same way. It is only the details of how he lived and how he died that distinguish one man from another – Ernest Hemingway

I sincerely hope you have found this book to be helpful in your pursuit of a dental practice. I'm truly honored to have provided you with my advice, learnings, and resources towards your vision.

My aspirations for writing this book as well as building the FirstTimeDentist.com website was driven solely off of you, the prospective practice owner. As I said earlier in the book, I went through this exact process in awe. Awe of how anyone could buy a dental practice, given the limited resources and questionable advisors I ran across during my wife's pursuit. My mission is to "*To INSPIRE practice ownership through ACTION.*"

As you have probably noticed, I have made quite a few notable mentions of the FirstTimeDentist.com website (perhaps too many!). I have, like you, high aspirations of making this website THE go to source for credible, trustworthy information – regarding a practice purchase and management.

Here is a brief glimpse of my plans for this website:

1. Blog / YouTube Content
2. Video Courses
3. Practice Calculators
4. Financial Tools / Advice.
5. E-Books
6. Podcasts
7. Mastermind Groups
8. Analysis Services
9. Demographic Tools
10. Personalized Coaching

In the end, I will not proclaim that I know everything there is to know about buying a practice. Quite the contrary, as I have always viewed myself as a student. To me, an expert is someone who is a perpetual student. Someone who is willing to subscribe to a lifestyle of continuous improvement and on-going learning. My methods, my approach, and even parts of my advice may adjust as I learn and experience more over time. However, I am convinced this is part of the process of building anything great.

As my middle school art teacher Mr. Wilkinson told us – "no piece of art is ever complete, the artist just doesn't know what the next step is."

With that, I want to leave you with a phenomenal quote that I have had hanging on my wall for quite some time. I refer to often as a way to keep life in perspective...

"To Laugh Often and Much
To win the respect of intelligent people and the affection of children
To earn the appreciation of honest critics and endure the betrayal of false friends
To leave the world a bit better; whether by a healthy child, a garden patch, or a redeemed social condition
To know that even one life has breathed easier because you have lived
This is to have succeeded"

                                          –RALPH WALDO EMERSON

My parting advice – it is not all about money. Business is about people, relationships and delivering superb a service/product which enhances your patients or customers life. The difference between poor and average is usually knowledge, but the difference between average and great is effort. I thank you again for purchasing this book and wish you the absolute best of luck in all your endeavors.

Should you have any feedback, questions, or comments – please feel free to visit FirstTimeDentist.com/contact.

Most Sincerely,

Adam Heim

ABOUT THE AUTHOR

Adam Heim has a diverse set of business experience and interests fused with an accomplished tenure in the corporate world of banking and finance. He started his career in deposit pricing optimization at several regional banks and then moved into branch and ATM distribution. In this role, he developed long-term strategic plans for the physical distribution network. Doing so required a deep understanding of financial modeling, customer behaviors / impacts, and commercial real estate.

Additionally, he has completed due diligence on multiple companies for the purpose of Mergers and Acquisitions at the bank. Adam has worked closely with a team of data scientists to build and refine a location analytics model (heatmap) for bank branch locations.

Throughout his experience in the corporate world, Adam Heim has also been building his industry knowledge in the dental field through the due diligence and eventual acquisition of his wife's dental practice in Southern Ohio in 2014. He has immersed himself in several entrepreurial endeavors which included residential real estate as well as FirstTimeDentist.com.

Adam resides with his wife, Amy, in their home in Southern Ohio. Adam spends his free time working on home renovation projects, gardening, cooking, hunting, riding ATVs and spending time in the great outdoors. Both Adam and Amy are life-long residents of the State of Ohio and enjoy the peace and tranquility which comes with living in a smaller town in a more rural setting.

END NOTES

i **Uncomplicate Business**: All It Takes is People, Time, and Money" (2015): Howard Farran; http://amzn.to/2rJElPk
ii **Checklist Manifesto: How to Get Things Right**" (2011): Atul Gawande; https://amzn.to/2IO07Zj
iii **"Will Smith – Face Your Fears"** (2017): Matesuz M: https://www.facebook.com/themateuszm/videos/1267997353298209/https://www.facebook.com/themateuszm/videos/1267997353298209/
iv **"Start with Why"** (2013): Simon Sinek TED Talk; https://youtu.be/sioZd3AxmnE
v **Who Moved My Cheese?** (1998): Spencer Johnson; http://amzn.to/2he30ZK
vi **"Warren Buffet's Rule of Thumb on Personal Integrity"** (2009): Nagesh Belludi; http://www.rightattitudes.com/2009/04/30/warren-buffett-on-personal-integrity/
vii **The 4-Hour Workweek: Escape 9-5, Live Anywhere, and Join the New Rich** (2009): Tim Ferris; http://amzn.to/2gpS5rS
viii **The E-Myth Revisited: Why Most Small Businesses Don't Work and What to Do About It** (2004); https://amzn.to/2pHkj8q
ix **The Power of Habit: Why We Do What We Do in Life and Business** (2014): Charles Duhigg; http://amzn.to/2hjGXyH
x **Ego is the Enemy** (2016): Ryan Holiday; http://amzn.to/2gBfxpm
xi **The Power of Vulnerability** (2011): Brene Brown; https://www.youtube.com/watch?v=iCvmsMzlF7o
xii **Small Business Administration**; www.sba.gov
xiii **Bank of America – Practice Solutions**; http://www.bankofamerica.com/practicesolutions
xiv **ESRI Business Analyst Online**; http://www.esri.com/software/businessanalyst/free-trial
xv **City-Data** – Advameg; www.City-Data.com
xvi **United States Census Bureau**; www.census.gov
xvii **ESRI**; http://www.esri.com/products/buyreports
xviii **Dentagraphics**; www.dentagraphics.com
xix **Zillow**; www.zillow.com
xx **Evernote**; www.evernote.com
xxi **"The Value of Goodwill"** (2015): Frank Brown (Dental Economics); http://www.dentaleconomics.com/articles/print/volume-105/issue-2/practice/the-value-of-goodwill.html

[xxii] **BusinessDictionary**; http://www.businessdictionary.com/definition/due-diligence.html
[xxiii] **"The Differences Between Financial Accounting and Management Accounting"** K.A. Francis (Chron); http://smallbusiness.chron.com/differences-between-financial-accounting-management-accounting-3985.html
[xxiv] **Google**; www.google.com
[xxv] **Internal Revenue Service**; https://www.irs.gov/businesses/small-businesses-self-employed/limited-liability-company-llc
[xxvi] **"Piercing the Corporate Veil"** (2016): Aaron Larson (ExpertLaw); https://www.expertlaw.com/library/business/corporate_veil.html
[xxvii] **"Why You Might Chose S Corp Taxation for Your LLC"**: Stephen Fishman (Nolo); http://www.nolo.com/legal-encyclopedia/why-you-might-choose-s-corp-taxation-your-llc.html
[xxviii] **Professional Solutions Insurance Company** (PSIC) ; https://www.psicinsurance.com/dentists/malpractice-insurance/program-highlights/default.aspx
[xxix] **"Letter of Intent Law and Legal Definition"**: US Legal https://definitions.uslegal.com/l/letter-of-intent/
[xxx] **National Plan & Provider Enumeration System (NPPES)**; https://nppes.cms.hhs.gov/#/
[xxxi] **U.S. Department of Justice**: Drug Enforcement Agency; https://www.deadiversion.usdoj.gov/

www.ingramcontent.com/pod-product-compliance
Lightning Source LLC
Chambersburg PA
CBHW031632210526

45464CB00004B/1861